Educators of Healthcare Professionals

Agreeing a Shared Purpose

Julie Browne, Alison Bullock,
Samuel Parker, Chiara Poletti,
John Jenkins, and Derek Gallen

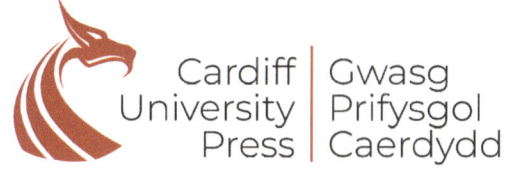

Published by
Cardiff University Press
Cardiff University
PO Box 430
1st Floor, 30–36 Newport Road
Cardiff CF24 0DE
https://cardiffuniversitypress.org

Text © Julie Browne, Alison Bullock, Samuel Parker, Chiara Poletti, John Jenkins and Derek Gallen 2021

First published 2021

Cover design by Hugh Griffiths
Front cover image: iStock.com/FatCamera

Print and digital versions typeset by Siliconchips Services Ltd.

ISBN (Paperback): 978-1-911653-24-0
ISBN (PDF): 978-1-911653-28-8
ISBN (EPUB): 978-1-911653-25-7
ISBN (Mobi): 978-1-911653-26-4

DOI: https://doi.org/10.18573/book6

This work is licensed under the Creative Commons Attribution-NonCommercial-NoDerivs 4.0 International License (unless stated otherwise within the content of the work). To view a copy of this license, visit http://creativecommons.org/licenses/by-nc-nd/4.0/ or send a letter to Creative Commons, 444 Castro Street, Suite 900, Mountain View, California, 94041, USA. This license allows for copying any part of the work for personal but not commercial use, providing author attribution is clearly stated. If the work is remixed, transformed or built upon, the modified material cannot be distributed.

The full text of this book has been peer-reviewed to ensure high academic standards. For full review policies, see https://cardiffuniversitypress.org/site/peer-review-policies/

Suggested citation:
Browne, J., Bullock, A., Parker, S., Poletti, C., Jenkins, J., and Gallen, D. 2021. *Educators of Healthcare Professionals: Agreeing a Shared Purpose*. Cardiff, UK: Cardiff University Press. DOI: https://doi.org/10.18573/book6. License: CC-BY-NC-ND

To read the free, open access version of this book online, visit https://doi.org/10.18573/book6 or scan this QR code with your mobile device:

Contents

List of Tables	v
List of Figures	vii
Acknowledgments	x
Contributors	xi
Foreword	xv
Chapter 1. Interprofessional Education: An Overview	**1**
Rationale and Background to the HEVA Study	11
Chapter 2. Phase 1: The Initial Survey	**17**
Method	17
Survey Results	18
Conclusions	24
Chapter 3. Phase 2: Analysis of Standards and Guidance Documents	**27**
Methods	27
Analysis of Documents	28
Findings	30
Summary and Conclusions	33
Chapter 4. Phase 3: The Nominal Group	**39**
The Nominal Group Process	39
The Participants	39
Results	40
Final Remarks	47
Chapter 5. Phase 4: Workshop	**49**
Methods	49
Results	50

Chapter 6. Phase 5: The Delphi Study — 71

The Delphi Process — 71
Overview of the Rounds — 72
The Participants — 72
Round 1 Results — 73
Round 2 Results — 89
The Final Consensus — 92

Chapter 7. Conclusions — 95

Limitations — 95
Conceptualising Generic DVAs — 96
Organisational Structure — 100
Final Domain Groupings — 101

Chapter 8. The Way Forward — 105

The Complexities of Interprofessional Teaching and Learning — 106
How a Common Framework Can Lead to Educational Improvements — 111
An Early Start to Educator Identity Development — 111
The Basis for Educational Excellence — 112
AFTERWORD: The Future of Interprofessional Education — 114

References — 117
Appendix 1: List of Standards Documents Analysed — 129
Appendix 2: Definition of Initial Codes — 137
Appendix 3: Coding Frequency for All Nodes — 147
Appendix 4: List of Abbreviations — 149
Index — 153

List of Tables

1. List of codes used in document analysis	29
2. Coding of professional values (number of documents = 48)	31
3. Coding of professional activities (number of documents = 38)	32
4. Initial values and modifications	42
5. First round voting	43
6. Second round voting	44
7. Initial activities list and modifications	45
8. First round voting	46
9. Second round voting	47
10. Items grouped as values	51
11. How Group 1 ordered the items	54
12. How Group 3 ordered the items	58
13. How Group 4 ordered the items	60
14. How Group 5 ordered the items	62
15. How Group 6 ordered the items	64
16. How Group 7 ordered the items	66
17. How Group 8 ordered the items	68
18. How Group 9 ordered the items	70
19. Round 1 results for values, ordered by mean	75
20. Round 1 comments about the values	76
21. Round 1 activities results for preparation for teaching and learning, ordered by mean	77
22. Round 1 comments on preparation of teaching and learning	79
23. Round 1 activities results for teaching and supporting learning, ordered by mean	80

24. Round 1 comments on teaching and supporting learning — 81
25. Round 1 activities results for learner progression, ordered by mean — 82
26. Round 1 comments on learner progression — 83
27. Round 1 activities results for working in teams, ordered by mean — 84
28. Round 1 comments on working in teams — 85
29. Round 1 activities results for enhancing quality, ordered by mean — 86
30. Round 1 comments on enhancing quality — 87
31. Round 1 results: Activities – Final comments — 88
32. Value included in second round — 88
33. Activities included in second round — 88
34. Round 2 results for value 'Interprofessional education' — 90
35. Activities results Round 2 (Round 1 results) — 90
36. Values achieving consensus after two rounds — 92
37. Activities achieving consensus after two rounds — 92

List of Figures

1. Role of educators – survey results for Q1. Do you teach, support or regulate the learning of health or social care professionals? (n=126)   18
2. Professionals whom respondents teach, support or regulate   19
3. Professional organisation membership: survey results for Q2. Do you teach, support or regulate the learning of health or social care professionals? (n=126)   20
4. Professional organisation membership – details.   20
5. Responsibility to a regulatory body: survey results for Q3. Are you responsible to a regulatory body for your personal professional practice? (n=126)   21
6. Regulatory bodies to which respondents are responsible   22
7. Professional practice as an educator appraised against standards: survey results for Q4. Is your personal professional practice as an educator evaluated or appraised against standards? (n=126)   22
8. Standards used to appraise professional practice as an educator   23
9. Use of other standards to guide professional practice as an educator: survey results for Q5. Are there any other standards or guidelines for educators of health or social care professionals that guide your practice? (n=126)   23
10. Other standards used to guide professional practice as an educator   24
11. Coding by document (Max no. codes = 42)   34
12. Coding comparison between the COPDEND Professional Standards for Dental Educators (Committee of Postgraduate Dental Deans and Directors 2013) and the Nursing and Midwifery Council Standards to Support Learning and Assessment in Practice (2008)   36

13. Coding comparison between Redressing the Balance (Academy of Medical Sciences 2010) and the College of Social Work Practice Educator Professional Standards for Social Work (2013) — 37
14. Overview of frequency of distribution of values and principles — 51
15. Group 1 worksheet — 55
16. Group 2 worksheet — 56
17. Group 3 worksheet — 57
18. Group 4 worksheet — 59
19. Group 5 worksheet — 61
20. Group 6 worksheet — 63
21. Group 7 worksheet — 65
22. Group 8 worksheet — 67
23. Group 9 worksheet — 69
24. Affiliations of Round 1 Delphi group participants — 73
25. Delphi group Round 1 rating of values — 75
26. Delphi group Round 1 rating of Activities 1 – Preparation for teaching and learning — 78
27. Delphi group Round 1 rating of Activities 1 – Teaching and supporting learning — 80
28. Delphi group Round 1 rating of Activities 3 – Learner progression — 82
29. Delphi group Round 1 rating of Activities 4 – Working in teams — 84
30. Delphi group Round 1 rating of Activities 5 – Enhancing quality — 86
31. Delphi group Round 2 rating of values — 90
32. Delphi group Round 2 rating of activities — 91
33. The descriptors of the 9 values and 24 activities, organised by domain — 102
34. How the DVA framework supports continuous quality improvement — 103
35. How the DVA framework supports educator progression — 104
36. Educator from profession A teaches learner or learners from profession A — 107

37. Educator from profession A teaches learner or learners from professions A and B 108
38. Educator from profession A teaches learner or learners from professions B and C 109
39. Educators from professions A, B and C teach learners from professions A, B and D 110

Acknowledgments

This study was supported by grants from Health Education and Improvement Wales HEIW and Health Education England HEE. We are grateful for this funding, which enabled us to undertake this study.

The work was informed by input from our advisory group, who provided critical feedback throughout.

Numerous participants have contributed to this study. Their contribution has been central, and we are most thankful for the time and energy they have put to critically engaging with drafts of the values and activities. We are particularly grateful to David Smith, Director of Strategy and Operation in INHWE (International Network for Health Workforce Education).

Contributors

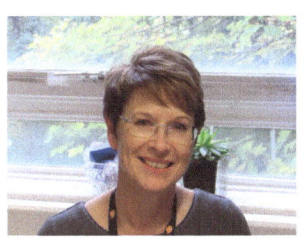

Julie Browne PGCE, MA, FacadMEd, SFHEA

Julie is a Senior Lecturer in Academic Practice at Cardiff University. In 2015 she was awarded the President's Silver Medal of the Academy of Medical Educators for outstanding and sustained contributions to medical education. Her professional background is in academic publishing, and she was Managing Editor of *Medical Education* and *The Clinical Teacher* from 2001 to 2008; she is currently Co-Chair of Cardiff University Press Editorial Board and Honorary Editor of *The British Student Doctor Journal*. She has been prominent in a number of national initiatives to improve the training and recognition of professional healthcare educators: a founding member of the Academy of Medical Educators, she currently serves as its Vice-Chair of Council.

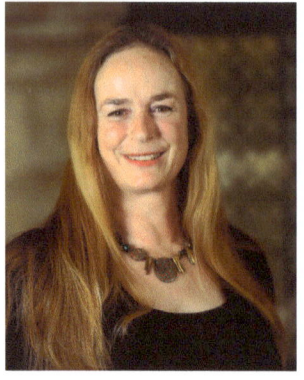

Alison Bullock PhD, FAcMedEd, PGCE, BA

Alison is Professor of Medical and Dental Education at Cardiff University, School of Social Sciences and, since 2009, Director of the Cardiff Unit for Research and Evaluation in Medical and Dental Education. The purpose of the Unit and her main activity is to conduct multidisciplinary research and evaluation of the education and training of healthcare professionals. She accumulated over 100 peer-reviewed publications and is Associate Editor of the *European Journal of Dental Education*. The other main aspects of her role include grant capture, doctoral supervision and research ethics committee work.

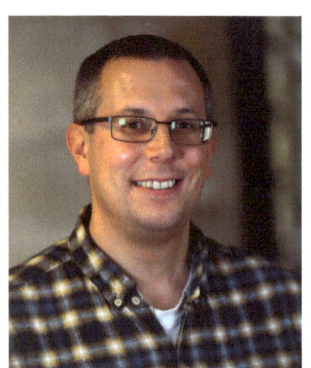

Samuel Parker PhD

Samuel completed his PhD in the School of Social Sciences, Cardiff University, in 2018. He is currently a Lecturer in Psychology at Birmingham City University, where he teaches courses in Qualitative Research Methods and Social Psychology.

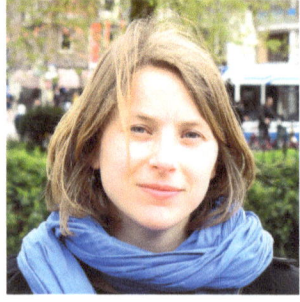

Chiara Poletti

Chiara is a PhD student at Cardiff University, School of Social Sciences (SOCSI). Since 2018, she has collaborated with the Cardiff Unit for Research and Evaluation of Medical and Dental Education (CUREMeDE), Cardiff University, working as Research Assistant on different projects, including the Educators of Healthcare Professionals: Shared Values and Activities Study (HEVAS) project, funded by Health Education England and the Wales Deanery at Health Education and Improvement Wales. She has also undertaken a review of research into health and care professional regulation since 2011, commissioned by the Professional Standards Authority (PSA), and is currently working on a scoping review of Out of Programme (OOP) schemes in the UK.

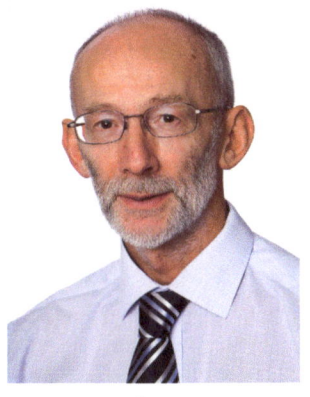

John Jenkins CBE MD (Hons) Hon.FRCPCH FRCP(Edin) FRCPI Hon.FAcadMEd

John is Honorary Professor, RCSI Healthcare University. He has been actively involved in the regulation, development and delivery of medical and interprofessional education in the United Kingdom and Ireland throughout his career as Consultant Paediatrician and Senior Lecturer in Child Health at Queen's University Belfast. Subsequently, since retirement he has been President of the Association for the Study of Medical Education and is independent Chair of the Medical Intern Board of Ireland. He is also a member of the AMEE ASPIRE Board and deputy Chair of the panel for Recognition of Excellence in Curriculum Development.

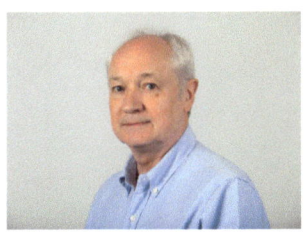

Derek Gallen FRCGP, FRCPE, MMEd, FHEA, FAcadMedEd

Derek is Professor Emeritus and is currently the president of the Association for the Study of Medical Education (ASME) and education lead for Medics Academy. He was previously the Postgraduate Medical Dean for Wales and UK National Director of the Foundation programme. He was a founding member of the Academy of Medical Educators and past President. He qualified as a general practitioner but moved into medical education at an early stage of his career. He has developed many innovative academic training programmes in the foundation years and is author of several books on general practice and medical education. His current research interests are in interprofessional education and assessments within postgraduate curriculum.

Foreword

The value of effective teamworking has become widely recognised in recent years, not only as a mechanism for better understanding between healthcare works but as making a significant contribution to a reduction in the number of avoidable errors. However, in many areas of healthcare delivery, the hierarchical approach is still in evidence due, in some part, to the way we train not only healthcare workers but the trainers themselves.

Learning one's own 'trade' can be difficult enough and many of us are content to restrict our teaching to the areas we know best. To be able to develop our teaching within the context of integrating those skills with the training and development needs of other professionals requires a real shift in mindset and approach. Understanding and valuing the learning requirements of other professions can be challenging at first, but the benefits to the learner, colleagues, patients and the wider healthcare workforce will be significant. On top of this, there are real personal benefits for the teacher and the teacher's development. Interprofessional learning is not just about sitting in the same room as professionals from other disciplines, and the teacher needs to be able to set up a structure which actively engages all groups in the overall learning process. A positive mindset needs to be built in at the early stages of a learner's development before set ways of working become ingrained, whilst recognising that the specific needs of individual professional groups also need to be met.

None of this can happen without careful planning by those delivering the learning, and this book sets out a manageable and consistent structure to support the planning and implementation of the interprofessional learning concept.

Interprofessional teaching offers an exciting challenge and a broad range of opportunities to those prepared to embrace it. The diversity of learning needs within an interprofessional group means that the teacher will have to develop a broader understanding of both the individual subject requirements and the areas of common ground across the groups. Gaining insight into the 'bigger picture' has the potential to further develop the teacher as well as the learner and to add real value to the teaching role.

The comprehensive and in-depth piece of work on which this book is based brings together existing scholarship and contemporary research to test a number of basic, but complex, areas and to refine these into a detailed manageable model which enables the teacher to develop a structured programme with the concept of shared values and activities at its heart. This results in an important practical approach that has the potential to make a significant contribution to improving quality and consistency in delivery of education and training to an interprofessional group.

The concept of the model is based on the identification of nine basic values that are fundamental to the delivery of quality-based, safe healthcare and the effective recognition of the importance of the individual and the co-worker in delivering care to patients. Delivery of these intrinsic values is supported by activities linked to four educational domains, which, through 24 structured areas, emphasise the importance of detailed teaching preparation to underpin the delivery of quality teaching, which, in turn, supports learning leading to progression of the learner and resulting in quality-assured educational activity and research.

This book will be of interest to all senior educators, education commissioners and managers, other educators looking to improve their educational practise or further develop their careers and a wide range of students interested in educational practice and practices. The content is not only applicable to the United Kingdom but will be of value to many of those involved in the development of quality-based interprofessional education models around the world.

Malcolm Smith
Postgraduate Dental Dean
Health Education England North East

CHAPTER 1

Interprofessional Education: An Overview

> Shaping safer organisations and teams is as important to patient safety as shaping safer practitioners. (Commission on Education and Training for Patient Safety 2016)

Spring 2017: nine senior officers from healthcare education societies and professional organisations across the United Kingdom meet in London to discuss the formation of a unified collaborative of healthcare education bodies.

Everyone is excited about the possibility of forming a federation of healthcare education organisations. There is a buzz in the air as discussions range around the potential for further collaboration, cross-recognition of members, sharing of resources, joint conferences, the development of genuinely interprofessional initiatives and even increased high-level influence. The meeting closes with warmth and goodwill on all sides and a decision to hold an online consultation, interviews with officers of key organisations and an associated number of 'town hall' meetings to see what the wider healthcare education community thinks of the idea.

But the report (ASME 2017) comes back with good news and bad news.

The good news is that the consultation response was overwhelmingly positive, with most of the 100-plus respondents welcoming closer collaboration and three quarters supporting the idea of a multiprofessional organisation to promote partnership working between healthcare education organisations.

The bad news is that few people really believe that collaboration can be achieved in practice. Everyone wants everyone to be involved, from educators of social workers, surgical trainers and hospital chaplains, but very few respondents actually think it can be done. Apart from the obvious practical issues relating to having to involve every healthcare education organisation

---

How to cite this book chapter:
Browne, J., Bullock, A., Parker, S., Poletti, C., Jenkins, J., and Gallen, D. 2021. Interprofessional Education: An Overview. *Educators of Healthcare Professionals: Agreeing a Shared Purpose.* Pp. 1–15. Cardiff, UK: Cardiff University Press. DOI: https://doi.org/10.18573/book6.a. License: CC-BY-NC-ND

in such a federation, and the perception that it wouldn't work if some professions were missing, the chief obstacles cited include traditional divides between professional groups, 'tribalism' and 'territorialism' between individuals and organisations and a belief that there is still insufficient interprofessional understanding regarding educator development, training roles and structures.

Something, it is clear, needs to be done.

The authors of this book firmly believe that this interprofessional understanding has to be worked out: it will not just emerge. But such an understanding cannot be achieved while each profession works independently to prepare training guidelines and standards for its own practitioners and focuses primarily on the education of its own professional group. Professions are, with some justification, proud of their own traditions. They cherish their individual expertise and knowledge, but the downside is that they may not value the expertise and knowledge of others. This book is therefore based on the firm conviction that the work of healthcare educators, regardless of profession, must be viewed holistically. For unless basic understandings of the work and attitudes of healthcare educators are developed interprofessionally from the outset, they risk being viewed – and rejected – as the 'property' of another profession.

We do not dispute that each healthcare profession has its own distinctive body of clinical knowledge. Those working in those professions, the practitioners – whether they be a mid-wife, a dentist or a physiotherapist, for example – develop their professional identities through exercising that clinical knowledge.

Our concern is for those who also perform educator roles, supervising trainees in the workplace, running educational programmes or lecturing undergraduates, for instance. Across healthcare professional groups, we know there is much in common in their educator roles, commonalities in terms of activities and values. Sadly, one key thing that healthcare educators share, regardless of profession, is that the role often lacks recognition. Throughout healthcare, there is a significant spectrum across professions in how education is viewed. At one extreme of the spectrum is a sense that developing a career as a healthcare educator is something for a small academic elite, destined to work full-time in a higher education establishment – and at the other extreme, that it is just an additional chore that clinicians have to do as part of their day job, requiring no additional skills or development. These competing discourses have a significant impact on the prevailing culture within the profession, which means that not all healthcare professions have guidelines for training their educators and those that do have variable standards and expectations, which can lead to misunderstanding and miscommunication between professions.

It is this problem, this lack of shared understanding and vision for the healthcare educator that led us to write this book. The research we undertook to underpin this publication has been a journey, focused on collecting evidence for a practical outcome, and one that we recount in the following chapters. We begin by elaborating the problem in this first chapter and set out our data gathering road map. In chapters 2 to 6 we report our empirical findings. In the final chapter we draw attention to some key debates we encountered and outline what emerged as a baseline framework of shared values and activities which can be used by all educators working in a health profession in planning their development as educators and gaining greater recognition for the role. The framework is also useful for managers and leaders of education as it establishes what can be expected of a healthcare educator at the outset of their career. We also argue that it sets the foundation for further work on setting out expectations of the more advanced education practitioner and for inter-professional educators. It is in the interest of all healthcare professions that their professional bodies work more closely together to consider how healthcare educators can be supported as a distinct body with unique expertise and skills.

The role of teams in patient safety

Clinical practice is an inherently high-risk environment. Around 1 in 10 hospitalised patients worldwide experiences some sort of adverse event, and it has been estimated that at least 50% of these were caused by preventable errors (World Health Organisation 2017). The evidence for the frequency of harm in primary care is more difficult to establish. Studies have put it as high as 24% although a scan of published research in 2011 suggested the actual figure is between 1 and 2% (The Health Foundation 2011). While this figure may appear low compared with the hospital data, it is important to remember that within NHS England, general practice alone provides over 300 million patient consultations each year (NHS England 2017). In other healthcare delivery environments, such as pharmacies, care homes and outpatient clinics, the figures for adverse events are even harder to establish, but the enormous numbers involved would suggest that even a low level of error would represent a significant amount of suffering and distress.

Adverse events have traditionally been viewed as the result of individual human action or inaction. The focus has been on the individual practitioner who causes harm due to factors affecting concentration and performance such as high workload, cognitive overload, failure of oversight, declining performance due to age, illness or substance dependency and so on; or in some rare cases, active malfeasance. The findings of the influential report *To Err is Human* two decades ago, however, caused organisations and individuals across the world to reassess this perspective (Institute of Medicine 2000). It concluded that:

> Current responses to errors tend to focus on the active errors. Although this may sometimes be appropriate, in many cases it is not an effective way to make systems safer. If latent failures remain unaddressed, their accumulation actually makes the system more prone to future failure. (Institute of Medicine 2000: 66)

Comparisons of healthcare's safety management systems with those of other high-risk sectors such as air travel and nuclear power have revealed significant differences in the way risk is viewed (Kapur et al. 2015; Reason 2000). In aviation it has long been recognised that preventable adverse outcomes are often the result of the failure of a whole team or system to avert a series of small mishaps that accelerate and accumulate until a catastrophic failure is caused (Vincent, Taylor-Adams & Stanhope 1998). Moreover, it is increasingly argued that focussing on the actions of the individual who made the most obvious error that occasioned the harm breeds a culture of blame, and this is not only distressing and psychologically traumatic for the individual to cope with but may lead to concealment, defensiveness or lack of acceptance of responsibility (Archer et al. 2017; Kirkup 2015). Albert Wu, introducing the concept of the second victim, suggests that those who make mistakes may often suffer devastating grief, distress and shame that effectively makes them victims of the same initial error that caused harm to the patient. One role of the team, he argues, is to help to 'make it feel safe to talk about mistakes' as a way of increasing learning about adverse events and reducing the damaging effect of the institutional marginalisation and isolation of colleagues who have made errors (Wu 2000). Litigation is a notoriously ineffective way to deal with error. Confession, restitution and absolution are essential to coping psychologically with the guilt of medical error, but when blame cultures prevail, lawyers and institutions may actively try to prevent practitioners from admitting an error. Blocking, or at least delaying this process, legal and institutional responses deprive colleagues of an early opportunity to confess their mistake, face up to the error, apologise and make restitution (Wu 2000). Worst of all, directing litigation towards the individual will not address the system failures that allowed the error to occur (Dekker 2013).

This refocussing of perspective on medical and healthcare error has led to a recognition within healthcare of the crucial importance of the role of teams in providing safe patient care (Reason 2000).

When teams fail to work together

There is a relationship between patient safety and the wider healthcare team. The catastrophic failures at Mid Staffordshire NHS Foundation Hospital Trust in the United Kingdom led to significant harm caused to individual patients by individual healthcare workers. But the Public Inquiry finding (see Francis 2013) was emphatic that these harms were the collective responsibility of the wider healthcare team. Harm to patients resulted from many failures of communication and teamworking through which a culture had developed that focused on numbers rather than people, avoidance of responsibility at all levels and too great a tolerance of poor standards (Francis 2013). The Department of Health response to the Francis report was clear about what needed to be done, and among its key recommendations it stated:

> Students and clinicians in training are the eyes and ears of the service today and the safety leaders of the future. They need to be trained not only in safe care of the patient in front of them – already central to training – but also in all the elements that are crucial to creating safer clinical systems: understanding human factors, measurement and audit, **effective multidisciplinary team working,** safe handovers of care, learning from errors and near misses, and the tools of improvement science. (Secretary of State for Health 2015: 28, authors' emphasis)

In 2014–15, partly in response to the public outrage as details of the events in Mid Staffordshire NHS Foundation Hospital Trust became known, the NHS introduced a legal requirement for duty of candour. Duty of candour is a statutory duty placed upon all NHS organisations and providers to be open and honest with patients and their families regarding adverse events, including alerting them to issues that may have caused or could cause significant harm, either now or in the future. This requirement is additional to the ethical responsibilities placed upon individual practitioners, and it reflects a realisation that less adversarial responses to error are needed (Powell 2020). Its main purpose is to reduce defensive behaviour by institutions who may, in the past, have been slow to reveal error, quick to blame and victimise individuals and strongly adversarial in defending their position (Birks et al. 2014). One of its key effects is to refocus the emphasis on the role of the whole multiprofessional healthcare team in taking responsibility for patient safety.

Everyone in the healthcare team has a responsibility to work effectively together to detect, analyse, treat and resolve a clinical challenge. While individuals may still make errors, effective teams work together to prevent those errors from escalating, and most importantly, will address the causes of those errors to ensure that they do not happen again. Lingard (2012), discussing the idea of collective competence, points out that teams are highly dynamic sub-systems within a complex and constantly changing healthcare system. Levels of team competence may fluctuate from moment to moment because healthcare is a 'constantly evolving set of multiple, interconnected behaviours enacted in time and space' in which team members are constantly learning through experience (Lingard 2012: 55). The force that holds all of these elements within the system in balance – individuals, the equipment they use, the norms under which they work, their collective understanding of what their objectives are, their social groupings and the way they divide up the work between them – is social communication (Engeström 1987).

Why do healthcare teams fail to work effectively together? The reasons are, of course, multiple, but the basic cause is almost always to do with a lack of effective communication (Foronda et al. 2016; Lingard et al. 2017). There are a number of factors that can affect how people communicate within teams. Sutcliffe et al. (2004), in an interview study involving 26 residents in a US teaching hospital, found that communication failures were not simply a matter of failure to impart or receive information; that many of these failures arose from more complex social causes such as:

> vertical hierarchical differences, concerns with upward influence, role conflict and ambiguity, and struggles with interpersonal power and conflict.

Sutcliffe and colleagues' results showed that juniors were concerned about raising issues with seniors for fear of causing offence or from a desire not to appear incompetent (2004). Sometimes they did not speak up simply because they felt that the other person was not open to communication. These issues, in which junior members of the team feel unable to speak up, are exacerbated where the senior/junior divide also involves different professions.

In addition to the communication challenges caused by 'vertical' lines of hierarchy, there may also be 'horizontal' issues between professional groups; even where team members are of relatively equal standing, challenges to good communication such as territorialism, prejudice, stereotyping, cultural misunderstandings and so on may still exist (Chadaga, Villines & Krikorian 2016; Salas, Sims & Burke 2005). Weller (2012) outlines the effects of these on clinical decision making and patient safety within the wider healthcare team:

> Speaking up against a power gradient, or challenging a member of a different 'tribe' requires courage, and so poor decisions may go unchecked. (Weller 2012: 134)

Now that the detrimental effect of traditional hierarchies on teams has been so widely exposed as a critical factor in adverse events, it is time for a more participative and democratic approach to healthcare work. However, as Bleakley, Bligh and Browne (2011) remind us,

> This requires a wholesale change in attitudes towards teamwork, a climate change, as a basis to a practice change in the culture. (Bleakley, Bligh & Browne 2011: 122)

The educational imperative

The quotation 'every system is perfectly designed to produce the results it gets' has been attributed to a number of people: like every good aphorism it has been repeated so often that its origins have been lost – and it has been repeated so often because people perceive it to be true. The healthcare education system is, sadly, perfectly designed to produce the results it gets.

Professionals learn how to practise during their basic education; at university, at college, in the hospital and clinical placement setting and in the community.

At the same time, they learn to act towards other professionals and patients in the ways they are shown how to act. So if they are not exploring, valuing and adopting innovative ways to work more effectively with other professionals, it is because they are not having the learning experiences that would produce this effect.

It follows that if patient safety is to become embedded within a more democratic, collaborative and candid approach to interprofessional communication and teamwork, then the education must change to produce this effect. And in order to change educational practice, you need to start with the teachers.

Many practical, wise and evidence-based solutions have been proposed to improve team working to enhance patient safety (Lark, Kirkpatrick & Chung 2018; McFadden, Stock & Gowen 2006). Efforts in recent years have been intense, and there have been numerous papers and reports advocating, reporting and evaluating patient safety initiatives such as the use of checklists, safety conferences, simulation, handover briefings, total quality improvement, toolkits, reporting systems and so on (Gandhi, Berwick & Shojania 2016). The clinical skills centre has become a hub for interprofessional team-based simulation, and the evidence is increasing regarding its efficacy as an effective education tool (Barleycorn & Lee 2018; Foronda, MacWilliams & McArthur 2016). Some 25 journals are currently published on the theme of patient safety, some of which have an explicit focus on the role of the wider healthcare team (National Center for Biotechnology Information 2020). Suggestions for practical solutions to improving team-based care for patients are numerous.

But whatever the proposed intervention aimed at improving team competence, they all have one thing in common. Their primary purpose will be to improve communication, and the mechanism by which improved communication will be achieved is always educational in nature. Staff need to be trained to work together in interprofessional teams to understand, implement and maintain any new procedure or technology, and it is invariably education that is recognised as the crucial factor in making possible the cultural changes needed to permanently embed the initiative (Argyris 1992). But to achieve good education, you need to ensure that you have good teachers, fully equipped and trained to ensure good learning and teaching.

Interprofessional education

The most frequently cited definition of interprofessional education (IPE) comes from the UK Centre of the Advancement of Interprofessional Education (CAIPE):

> Interprofessional education occurs when two or more professions learn with, from and about each other to improve collaboration and the quality of care. (Barr 2002)

The important part of this definition is, we argue, the phrase 'with, from and about'. Interprofessional education, it is clear from this expression, is not just a case of learners from diverse professional groups sitting passively side by side to learn the same material; such a learning experience is more accurately described as multiprofessional education. In interprofessional education, the students must actively engage with others from different professional groups as they learn with, from and about them – active, experiential, social learning is baked into the concept of interprofessionalism.

This presents enormous challenges for those who wish to 'amplify the heterogeneity of learning groups' as Della Freeth (2010) puts it. The practical difficulties surrounding resources, timetables, curricula, teaching estate, student readiness to learn interprofessionally, effects on professional identity and so on, have been well rehearsed (Hammick et al. 2007; Mladenovic & Tilden 2017). But before one can even begin to address the practical issues involved in teaching interprofessional groups, attention must be paid to the training needs of those who are expected to prepare, deliver, assess and evaluate interprofessional learning.

Interprofessional education, by its very nature, cannot be done by a single individual. It necessarily involves teams of teachers and facilitators to work together effectively to produce learning opportunities. Between them these educators must, among many other tasks, establish the learning needs for each professional group and ensure the relevance of content; identify whether IPE is the most effective and feasible method for teaching some things; understand where the learning will fit within the curriculum or agenda of each group; anticipate any technical, resource or timetabling challenges; and design a learning event that will meet the needs of all the learners – including introducing and enhancing the 'soft skills' of collaboration, communication, teamworking and understanding that IPE, done well, is so effective at developing.

In short, to do IPE well requires teachers and trainers who themselves are able to work effectively in an interprofessional team to develop learning opportunities for a diverse group of students.

Teaching in interprofessional teams

Teachers working to prepare interprofessional learning for students and trainees are automatically expected to work in teams. But if the previous discussion of patient safety and teamworking within healthcare tells us anything, it is that teamworking is an extremely complex undertaking that needs careful consideration, excellent communication and some basic shared understandings about the purpose and nature of what is to be done. For, as Lorelei Lingard observes:

1. Competent individuals can come together to form an incompetent team.
2. Individuals who perform competently in one team may not in another team.
3. One incompetent member functionally impairs some teams, but not others.
   (Lingard 2012: 44)

Moreover, the barriers that apply to healthcare teams' effective communication – tribalism, territorialism, hierarchies and power imbalances, prejudice and stereotyping – are just as likely to apply in interprofessional teaching teams as they are anywhere else. These barriers may be even more challenging when teaching teams include, as they frequently do, individuals from non-clinical backgrounds. Such non-clinical teachers may include academics from disciplines outside healthcare such as social and biomedical scientists, humanities scholars, administrators, technologists and, of course, simulated or expert patients, actors and real patients and their families and carers.

While the research literature calls repeatedly for improved staff development for those who will be delivering IPE, such training programmes are not common (Health Professions Network Nursing and Midwifery Office 2010: 17). Where they do exist, they are primarily aimed at an individual level and involve imparting knowledge and skills around the implementation of IPE; few specifically address the development of team competences or the need to overcome ingrained professional attitudes regarding educational practice that might obstruct effective teamworking (Baerg, Lake & Paslawski 2012).

How healthcare educators acquire their professional identity

The path to becoming a healthcare educator is rarely smooth, whatever the background. Not everyone who sets out to make the move from clinician (or other primary profession) to educator stays the course (Neese 2003; Sabel et al. 2014). While nearly all clinicians undertake clinical and workplace supervision, a much smaller number would actually describe themselves as teachers or educators or admit to an emotional attachment to their educational activities (Riveros-Perez & Rodriguez-Diaz 2017; Sabel et al. 2014). Recent studies into educator development are largely agreed on this point; becoming a healthcare educator involves a series of sometimes painful changes and transitions (Browne, Bullock & Webb 2018; Cantillon, Dornan & De Grave 2019). Throughout these changes the individual progresses from self-identifying predominantly with their professional group within healthcare (for example, dentist, nurse, occupational therapist) to acquiring and assimilating a further dimension to their identity – that of educator (Sethi et al. 2017).

There are many aspects to healthcare education that make this transition from clinician to clinician-educator difficult; frequently cited challenges include the pressures of clinical work, the perception that healthcare education is lower status than clinical practice, reward systems that continue to recognise excellence in research and clinical service while failing to appreciate excellence in teaching, unclear career paths and difficulties with accessing information and training (Hu et al. 2015; Steinert, O'Sullivan & Irby 2019). While these practical challenges are a deterrent, more work needs to be done to establish the root causes of this internal struggle with identity that so many healthcare educators experience, and we hypothesise that these may be as much to do with the way that healthcare professionals are educated and socialised as with any specific systemic issues.

Educational skills are rarely included as part of the core curriculum in undergraduate healthcare professions. There is a 'hidden curriculum' to this – because if students are never exposed to the idea that they must develop teaching skills as part of their skillset as professionals in healthcare, they will graduate from universities and training programmes unaware of the value and importance of education in maintaining and improving standards of healthcare (Hafferty & O'Donnell 2014; Amorosa, Mellman & Graham 2011). It is then a very long journey to acquiring the additional threshold concept that education is not supplemental to, but integral to, their practice as healthcare professionals.

The landscape of CPD as a healthcare professional

Although educators must make a difficult conceptual leap from clinician to clinician-educator, the process by which this happens takes place largely within the security of their own profession. Their first roles will involve them in teaching students and trainees from their own profession, alongside teachers from their own profession. When they decide they need more formal development, they will attend courses alongside other learners from their own profession (and in some professions they can even undertake specialised postgraduate qualifications in, for example, Nursing, Medical or Dental Education). They may join an association or organisation for education within their own profession, and they will read academic literature that focuses on the education of their own profession. Their first formal appointment as a teacher is likely to be within a university school or college of their own profession or as an educational supervisor of trainees in their own profession. Their values, experiences, knowledge and behaviours will come directly from their own profession's 'education tribe'. They will even acquire their own terminology – apparently neutral terms such as 'trainee', 'clinical supervisor', 'practice observation', 'academic mentor' and 'clinical assessor' may mean totally different things depending on which profession is using them. Their concepts of good education, and even their philosophical and theoretical perspectives may be subtly different.

The implications of this for interprofessional educators are obvious. If the transition from new graduate to educator is difficult to negotiate, the transition from educator to interprofessional educator – equipped with the knowledge, skills and experience to role model interprofessional collaboration and to work constructively within an interprofessional team to deliver IPE – is very nearly as great.

This is where the work we describe in this book begins. We argue that very little lasting improvement, in terms of skills development, working conditions, career progression and educational delivery at the grass roots, can take place without a fundamental consensus from across all professions about how good teachers can be developed, recognised, recruited and rewarded. The dream of truly integrated interprofessional education depends on team competence. Such competence needs to be based on shared values and understandings together with an equivalence of basic skills that cannot yet be taken for granted.

As we describe the large-scale project that we undertook to establish a consensus on a framework for outlining the basic skills and values that all healthcare educators share, we will show that many widespread and naturalised assumptions about the nature of healthcare education cannot be taken for granted. Our work has revealed some of the fundamental but hitherto hidden lines of commonality and divergence between professions: issues concerning the skills, knowledge and attitudes of the individual educator versus the team or the institution, lines of responsibility for education, even the intellectual and disciplinary traditions that have shaped healthcare education within professions. We hope to show that educators in healthcare have much in common, regardless of professional group. But at the same time, we will also challenge professional groups to reflect on their own approach to educator development and consider if they are really doing enough to support those who are seeking to develop their careers as advanced and interprofessional educators. We encourage them to look beyond the education of their own learners, students and trainees, to reflect on whether traditional territorial attitudes (that they may sincerely believe are a thing of the past) are lingering on in their educational structures and processes (Nancarrow & Borthwick 2005; Sevens & Reeves 2019).

Rationale and Background to the HEVA Study

Healthcare professions educator careers

While each profession has its own distinctive body of clinical knowledge and expertise, in educational terms there is much that all professions can share, and many areas in which they can learn from each other. Good teamwork is essential to safe and effective patient care. Evidence has steadily accumulated that a broader approach to the preparation of all healthcare professionals is critical to their effectively working together in the clinical environment, including through the identification and incorporation into curricula of relevant collective competences. It is therefore important to develop a common language in order to facilitate positive dialogues between and within healthcare professions educators and the organisations that represent them.

Interest in the scholarship, research, delivery and evaluation of UK healthcare education has also expanded greatly over the last 50 years. This has led to the formation of a number of learned societies and professional bodies, which have made great strides towards professionalising the education of healthcare professionals (HCPs). Healthcare education has rightly emerged as a complex, rigorous and rewarding discipline in its own right.

Despite this, healthcare educators (HCEs) continue to face severe challenges in their career development regardless of their primary discipline or specialty (Albert et al. 2007; Parrott, Lee & Markless 2017). Career paths remain unclear; training for the role is patchy; and information difficult to access (Bartle & Thistlethwaite 2014; Browne et al. 2018). Many HCEs report that teaching within their profession is considered low status, and excellent performance as a teacher is still viewed as less prestigious than success in research or commitment to clinical practice and service delivery (Darbishire, Isaacs & Miller 2020). Finding time and resources for teaching and professional development remains challenging and is likely to become more so as staffing and funding levels have not kept pace with demand for service. This applies both in the healthcare system and also in higher education. Finally, recognition for the role is often lacking, with supervisors and line managers reportedly unclear about how to appraise and reward excellence in an educational role (Bittner & Bechtel 2017; Cantillon et al. 2019).

Interprofessional learning

In recent years it has become apparent that a more collaborative approach to the professional development of healthcare educators is needed in response to the changes in healthcare that are taking place, in particular with regard to the rapid rise of inter- and multiprofessional team working. Interprofessional learning (IPL) is now a key part of undergraduate and postgraduate curricula, mandated by several educational regulators.

But while IPL is becoming a key part of the education of a new generation of HCPs, support and training for HCEs remains largely mono-professional. There are several learned societies that cut across professional divides (examples include CAIPE, ASPiH, EBMA, INHED) and these have contributed greatly to the development of an academic foundation for learning and working together effectively: but as yet they are additional to, not alternatives to, the big mono-professional bodies such as the Royal Colleges, which set curricula, and the smaller mono-professional learned societies and interest groups to which many HCEs belong.

As an example, significant challenges are currently faced by, say, nurse educators or doctors running professional development events for dental educators or physiotherapists. Each professional grouping may be doing a magnificent job, but each is working within a slightly different framework and may therefore have slightly different standards and understandings that arise from their individual professions' approach to the support of educators. The potential for misunderstanding and miscommunication is considerable; as IPL becomes more embedded, the risks are paradoxically greater because not all HCPs have open guidelines for training for their educators.

Professional bodies in healthcare education

It is in the interest of all HCPs that their professional bodies work more closely together to consider how HCEs can be supported as a distinct body with unique expertise and skills rather than as small and undervalued subsets of individual professions. Mergers, collaboratives and federations, grouped around a shared set of values and understandings, are a long overdue solution to raising the collective profile of all educators in whatever area of healthcare professions education they are working.

Healthcare education also needs a strong and united voice if it is to have the necessary influence at national level to provide evidence for and secure the priority and resourcing required to further develop the systems of education and training across the healthcare professions, which will be essential in order to achieve a vision for the United Kingdom. One way to facilitate and support this would be the development of closer relationships between all such organisations and the regulators of the relevant professions.

The purpose of this book and outline of data collection

The primary aim of the research that forms the central portion of this book is to identify, discuss and establish, using a fully interprofessional approach, shared key values regarding the purpose and practice of healthcare education and key areas of educational activity that would be relevant, acceptable and useful to a broad range of healthcare educators. Core parts of the evidence gathering and analysis were funded by Health Education England and the Wales Deanery at Health Education and Improvement Wales. As a guide to the chapters that follow, we provide an overview of the evidence gathering and analysis which was undertaken in five phases, each designed to build on the outcomes of the earlier phase(s).

We used consensus methods within a mixed-methods, iterative design, undertaking the study in five phases which each built on the outcomes of prior phases. In phase 1, we distributed an online survey to international healthcare educators (completed by 126 respondents from a wide range of professions). Individual demographic data such as names and emails, employing institutions or country of origin were not sought. Questions focussed on respondents' membership of professional organisations for educators and whether their educator practice is guided by standards or guidelines or appraised. Follow-up, free text questions asked respondents to provide further details about who they taught, the bodies to which they were responsible, and the standards documents by which their teaching practice was currently appraised and evaluated. As data were provided anonymously, consent for participation was indicated by check box.

Recruitment was primarily by social media with the aim of attracting as diverse a group of respondents as possible (King, O'Rourke & DeLongis 2014). A snowballing approach was taken to the distribution of the survey and included emailing the link to known educators, a general call through social media (Facebook and Twitter) together with requests to key organisations for retweets and the use of hashtags such as #clined, #nursed, #HCP etc. At a rough estimate the call received around 73.5K impressions (Twitter analytics). The survey was open for one month.

In phase 2, we used the responses of the respondents to the initial survey (phase 1) to help us identify standards and guidance documents. We also sourced documents from internet searches and from the websites of regulators and professional bodies. In total, we collated and analysed 48 international professional standards and guidance documents to identify key themes. The analysis of the documents from a range of health professions was conducted independently by two members of the research team using NVivo software to code values and activities. The Academy of Medical Educators' (AoME) *Professional Standards* (2014) was taken as the baseline for developing codes as this was the only document that claimed applicability to HCEs from more than one profession (medical, dental, physician associate and veterinary). A further 12 codes were added to the 30 codes derived from the AoME *Professional Standards* (including the seven principles of public life), which brought the total number of codes to 42 (21 professional values and 21 activities).

In phase 3, a nominal group meeting was held in which participants were presented with the outcomes of the phase 2 document analysis. A shortlist of 20 key experts in the field of healthcare was drawn up. These were purposively selected on the basis of: seniority; diversity of professional background; maximum experience of leadership in the broader healthcare setting (e.g., senior position within a multidisciplinary organisation); and maximum coverage of all four nations in the United Kingdom plus the Republic of Ireland. Eight senior clinical educators with significant educational leadership profiles within their professions agreed to take part in the one-day session; participant data were anonymised for reporting purposes.

Following discussion of key issues for their profession, the 21 values and the 21 activities identified in phase 2 were discussed and clarified in turn, resulting in the combination of some items and the addition of new items. Participants then voted on the items in the agreed list using six voting cards (two cards with three points; two cards with two points; and two cards with one point), privately assigning their votes to the six items they judged most important. The results were collated, displayed and discussed. Following further amendments, participants voted a second time. The second voting allowed participants to modify their choices in the light of the feedback. The results were recorded and displayed, and comments and discussion sought. Field notes of the discussions were taken by author Chiara Poletti and later reviewed by the research team.

Phase 4 was also based on the results of phase 2. The 21 values and 21 activities identified in phase 2 were used as the basis for a combined plenary presentation and workshop with about 90 European and international health professions educators. JB and JJ were invited by the International Network of Health Workforce Education (INHWE) in Dublin in January 2019 to present details of the project so far and to engage delegates in the project. Following a 30-minute plenary presentation outlining the purpose of the project, delegates were invited to form smaller groups and to use their skills and expertise to thematically arrange the list of 42 values and activities. Written consent was not sought from participants; delegates were assured that participation was voluntary and anonymous.

This assisted the final organisation of activities into broad themes.

The results of phases 3 and 4, when combined, enabled us to more effectively present the values and activities. The fifth and final phase was a two-round Delphi study (Chuenjitwongsa 2017; de Villiers et al. 2005) Participants were recruited through an open call on social media; consent forms were distributed by email and on receipt of these, links to the survey were provided. Healthcare educators from a broad range of professions took part (n=37 Round 1; n=32 Round 2) in a ranking exercise to establish which of nine values and 33 educator activities were essential, desirable, optional or not necessary. The values and activities were derived from the original 42 codes used in the document analysis (phases 1 and 2), partially modified in the light of the nominal group (phase 3) and grouped into sections in the light of the workshop (phase 4).

The study was reviewed and approved by a Cardiff University Research Ethics Committee. The project was viewed by the Committee as service evaluation not requiring ethical approval [Ref#18/19; email 21-03-2018]. This project was funded by Health Education England and the Wales Deanery at Health Education and Improvement Wales.

We provide further details on methods at the start of each section reporting the results.

CHAPTER 2

Phase 1: The Initial Survey

The main purpose of this initial survey was to find out about how healthcare professions educators engaged with professional standards and regulation. We were keen to collate information on the extent and variety of standards and guidance by which healthcare educators were appraised and regulated. We hoped that this very short survey would help us in our search for relevant standards and guidance. In this section we summarise the findings of the survey and provide details of the current standards by which educators of health and social care professionals are appraised and evaluated.

Method

A short survey consisting of five questions was created using Online Surveys. The five questions asked were:

1. Do you teach, support or regulate the learning of health or social care professionals?
2. Do you belong to a professional organisation for educators of health or social care professionals?
3. Are you responsible to a regulatory body for your personal professional practice?
4. Is your personal professional practice as an educator evaluated or appraised against standards?
5. Are there any other standards or guidelines for educators of health or social care professionals that guide your practice?

For each question, where respondents indicated a 'yes' response, a follow-up, free text question asked those completing the questionnaire to provide further details about who they taught, the bodies to which they were responsible, and

---

How to cite this book chapter:
Browne, J., Bullock, A., Parker, S., Poletti, C., Jenkins, J., and Gallen, D. 2021. Phase 1: The Initial Survey. *Educators of Healthcare Professionals: Agreeing a Shared Purpose.* Pp. 17–25. Cardiff, UK: Cardiff University Press. DOI: https://doi.org/10.18573/book6.b. License: CC-BY-NC-ND

the standards documents their teaching practice was currently appraised and evaluated by.

The link to the survey was distributed via email to project partners and on Twitter through the Academy of Medical Educators and CUREMeDE accounts. A snowballing approach to social media was taken with requests to key organisations for retweets and the use of hashtags such as #clined, #nursed, #HCP etc., garnering around 73.5K impressions (Twitter analytics). The survey was open for one month.

Survey Results

The survey was completed by 126 respondents who either teach, support or regulate the learning of health and social care professionals. Responses were not limited to educators in the United Kingdom and indeed educators in Ireland, Italy, Spain, Australia, Zambia, Zimbabwe, Canada and the United States of America completed the survey.

The great majority of respondents (90%) stated that they were actively involved in teaching. Among all respondent the biggest group (40%) stated that they teach health and social care professionals whilst 32% stated that they both teach and support health and social care professionals. Figure 1 further shows that 16% of respondents had a role in teaching, supporting and regulating the learning of health and social care professionals and that smaller numbers were also involved in supporting and regulating only. This reassured us that we had targeted the questionnaire at people who were working in the healthcare educa-

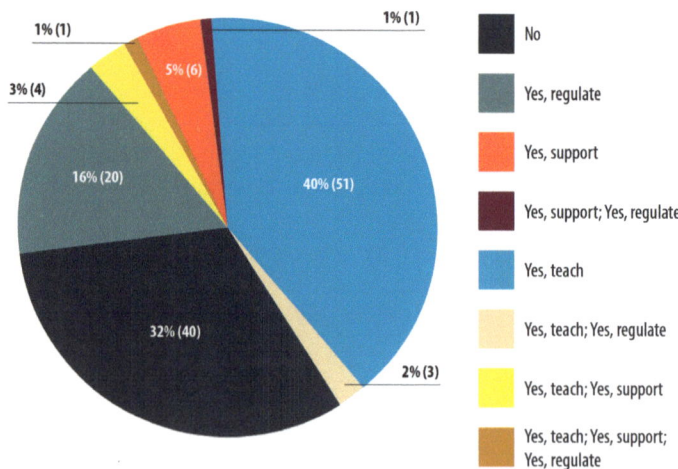

Figure 1: Role of educators – survey results for Q1. Do you teach, support or regulate the learning of health or social care professionals? (n=126)

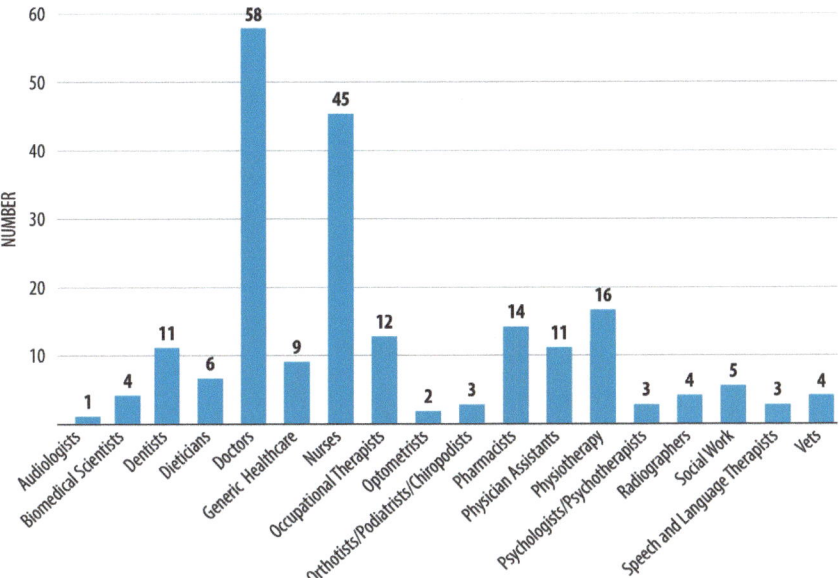

Figure 2: Professionals whom respondents teach, support or regulate.

tion context and thus would be aware of and affected by the education regulatory and professional context.

Figure 2 shows the wide range of professions who were consulted in this survey. Many respondents listed several professional groups that they teach which have been counted separately in Figure 2. Whilst respondents were most likely to teach, support or regulate the learning of doctors or nurses, there were also a good number of responses received from those who teach dentists, occupational therapists, pharmacists and physiotherapists. Although there were smaller numbers of respondents involved in the teaching, supporting and regulation of other professional groups (such as audiologists and optometrists), it was encouraging that such a wide range of professions took part in this consultation.

Question 2 asked respondents to indicate whether they belonged to a professional organisation for educators of health and social care professionals. Figure 3 shows that 61% of respondents did indeed belong to such an organisation. We deliberately left it to the respondents to decide what constituted a professional organisation for educators. Their responses showed a variety of different bodies ranging from employers, professional licensing bodies, national professional regulators and voluntary and advisory organisations, once again indicating the diversity and complexity of the professional landscape and the potential for multiple and potentially conflicting perspectives on education guidance and regulation, depending on memberships.

Those who answered 'yes' to this question were asked to state the organisations of which they were members. Responses are summarised in Figure 4.

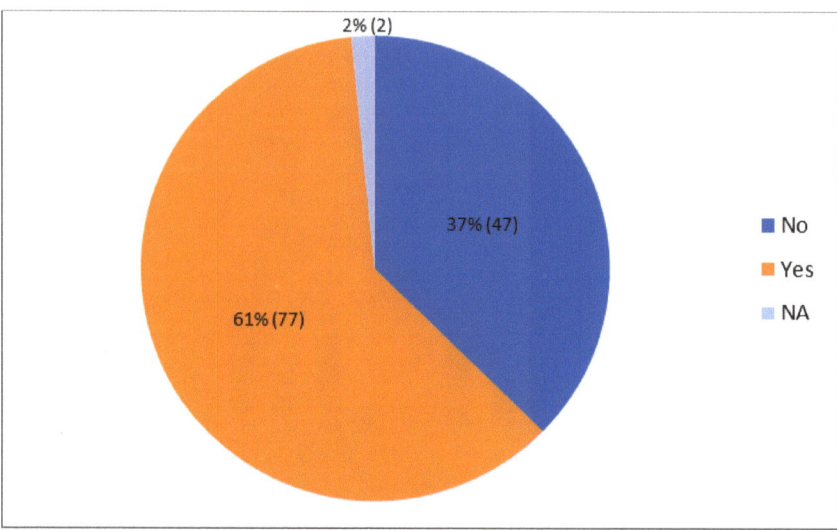

Figure 3: Professional organisation membership: survey results for Q2. Do you teach, support or regulate the learning of health or social care professionals? (n=126)

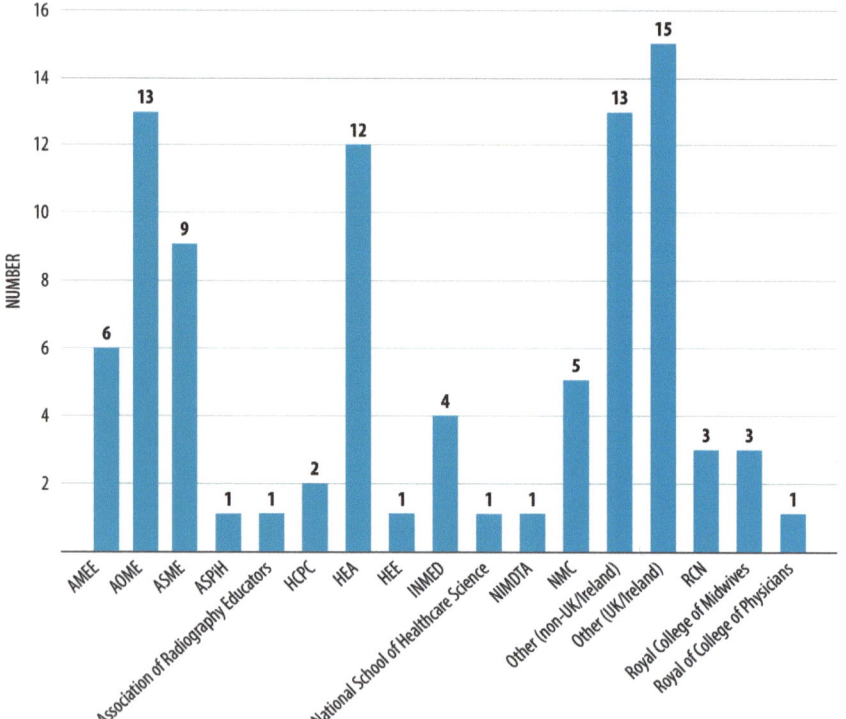

Figure 4: Professional organisation membership – details.

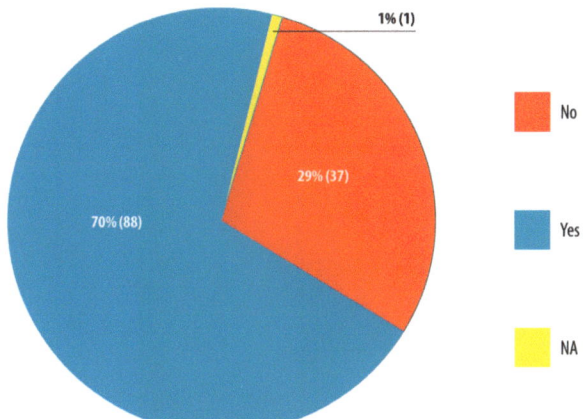

Figure 5: Responsibility to a regulatory body: survey results for Q3. Are you responsible to a regulatory body for your personal professional practice? (n=126)

A wide range of responses was received for this question with organisations such as the Academy of Medical Educators (13), the Association for the Study of Medical Education (9) and the Association for Medical Education in Europe (6) commonly given. The Higher Education Academy (12) was also an organisation to which several respondents belonged. A smaller number of respondents also listed being part of the key organisations shown in Figure 4 and also a number of smaller UK and overseas organisations that have been grouped together into 'other' columns in order to aid representation in the figure.

Whilst 61% of respondents reported belonging to an organisation for educators of health and social care professionals, Figure 5 shows that a slightly higher number of respondents (70%) indicated that they were responsible to a regulatory body for their personal professional practice. Figure 6 shows that the General Medical Council (24), Nursing and Midwifery Council (21) and Health and care Professions Council (18) were the organisations to whom the largest numbers of respondents were responsible. Again, however, there was a large number of different responses to this question given by respondents that have therefore been grouped as 'other' in this figure.

Despite 70% of respondents claiming to be responsible to a regulatory body for their personal professional practice, Figure 7 shows that only 59% had their educator practice appraised against a relevant set of standards or guidance.

As with previous questions, the free text follow-up to those who answered 'yes' to Question 4 revealed a range of standards against which educators' professional practice was appraised. Figure 8 shows that internal university standards (12), the Nursing and Midwifery Council Standards (11), Higher Education Authority and General Medical Council standards (10 each) and Academy of Medical Educators Standards (7) were the most commonly used standards for appraising the practice of educators.

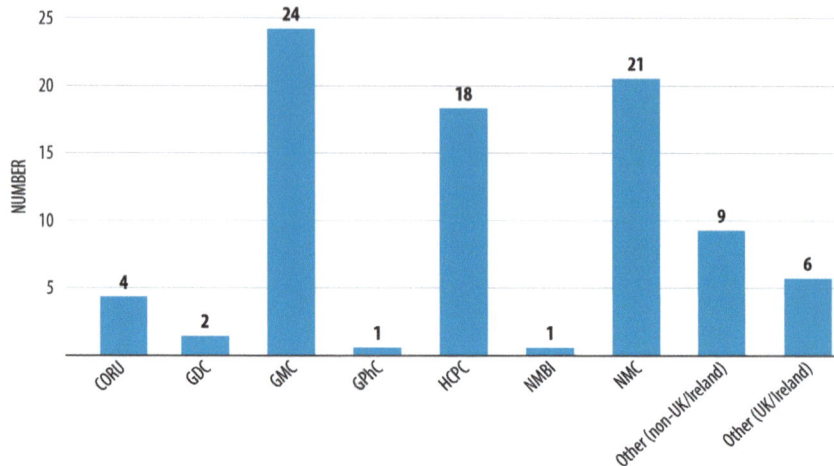

Figure 6: Regulatory bodies to which respondents are responsible.

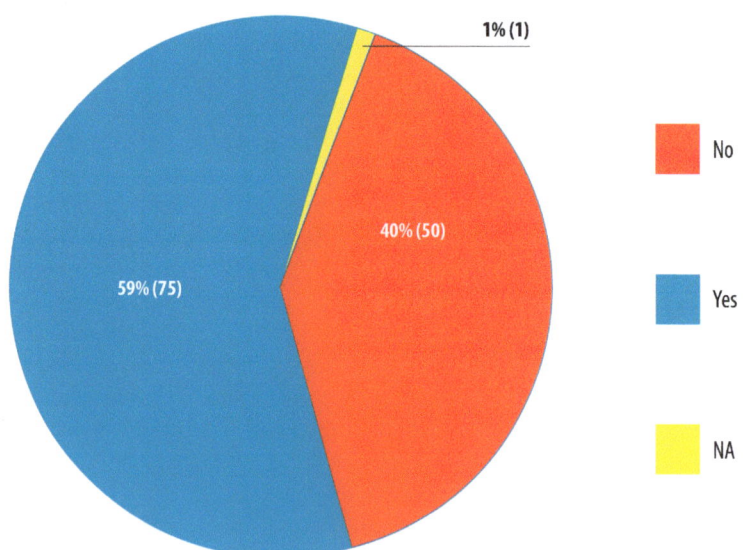

Figure 7: Professional practice as an educator appraised against standards: survey results for Q4. Is your personal professional practice as an educator evaluated or appraised against standards? (n=126)

Figure 9 shows that 56% (n=71) of respondents also referred to using other standards and guidelines in order to guide their professional practice, while Figure 10 gives details of which organisations' guidance was used.

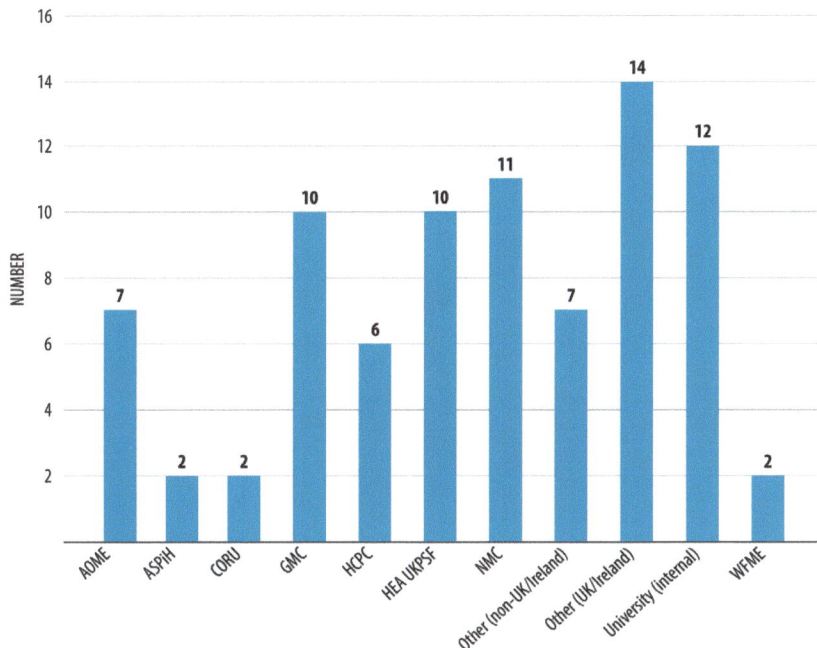

Figure 8: Standards used to appraise professional practice as an educator.

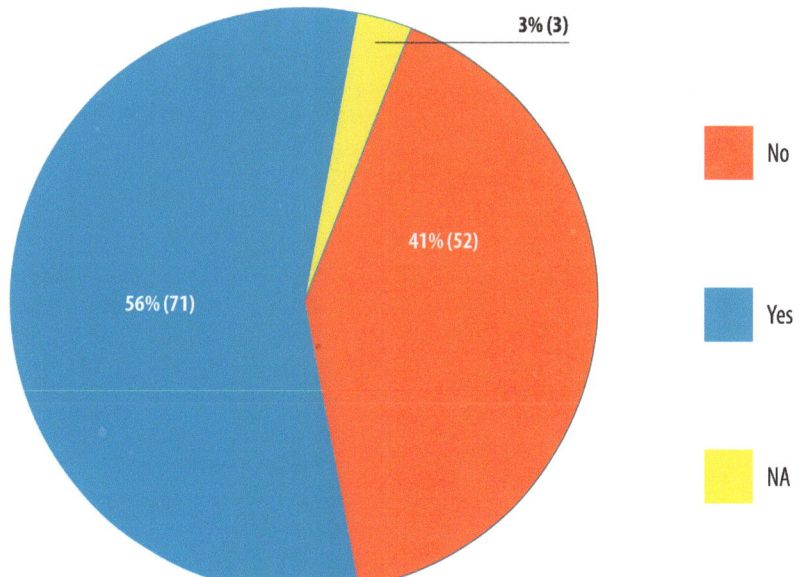

Figure 9: Use of other standards to guide professional practice as an educator: survey results for Q5. Are there any other standards or guidelines for educators of health or social care professionals that guide your practice? (n=126)

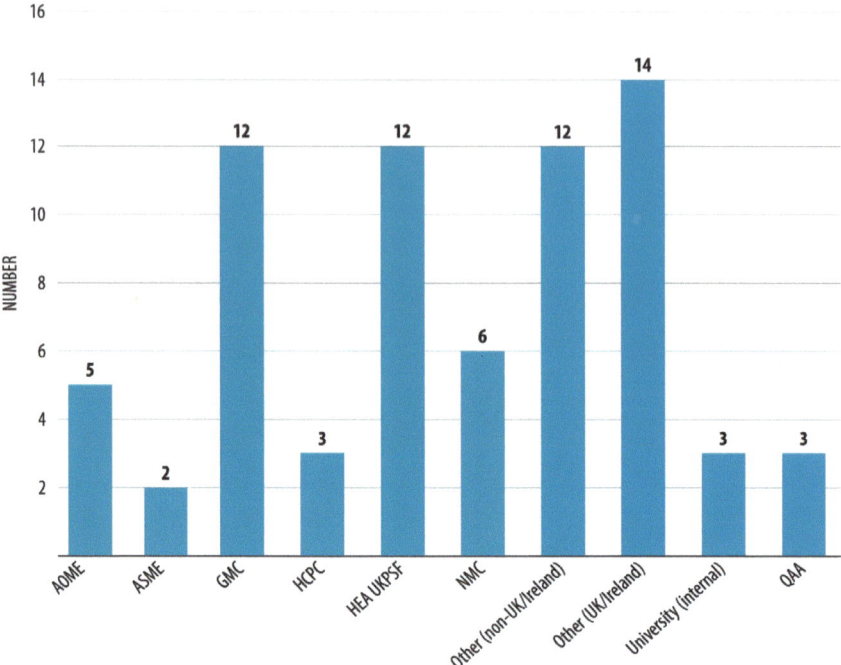

Figure 10: Other standards used to guide professional practice as an educator.

Unlike Question 4, in which university institutional guidelines were given as the most common standard for assessing professional practice, respondents indicated here that HEA and GMC guidelines (12 each), NMC (6) and Academy of Medical Educators standards were also used to guide their individual professional practice.

Conclusions

The purpose of this survey was to consult with a wide range of healthcare professions educators from different health and social care professions and to ascertain which standards healthcare professions educators are currently using to guide their professional practice as educators. We were particularly keen to know the degree to which respondents were aware of or made use of healthcare education standards and guidance and, if we could, to identify additional standards that our original search had not uncovered. As such, an additional aim of consulting with educators was to ensure that the mapping of standards documents and guidance, being undertaken as the first stage of the wider project, was as comprehensive as possible. We were pleased to be able to include in the first stage of data analysis an additional ten standards documents as a result of this consultation.

Educators from a wide range of professional backgrounds engaged with this consultation and the results of this survey reveal that there are a range of standards by which healthcare professions educators' practice is currently evaluated, but also that there are additional standards which further inform their practice. The relationship between these sets of standards and how they are understood, used and reconciled in individual cases needs further exploration. A medical educator, for example, may be aware of frameworks developed by his or her Trust, by Health Education England, the General Medical Council and voluntary organisations such as the Association for Simulated Practice in Healthcare or the Higher Education Academy (AdvanceHE) but we cannot yet say which guidance takes priority or is most relied upon by the individual practitioner.

CHAPTER 3

Phase 2: Analysis of Standards and Guidance Documents

Methods

Literature review

We performed an initial search for professional standards documents using internet search engines. As this was primarily a search for 'grey literature' – reports, guidance, policy statements and frameworks, a systematic review of research literature was not required. Within search engines (primarily PubMed, Bing and Google) and also regulator and professional organisations' websites, terms such as 'clinical educator', 'health professions education', 'values', 'guidance' and 'standards' were entered. This included searching for standards for healthcare professions educators in at least 25 professions, which were also added to the search terms. To ensure coverage of each profession a further search of the websites for regulators and societies of each of these professions was also undertaken. Search results were not limited to the United Kingdom and Ireland, although this was the focus of the research, in order to obtain as broad a consensus on shared values and activities as possible.

This initial literature search resulted in 44 documents being identified. Upon further reading of the documents it became clear that some were standards for individual healthcare professions educators (e.g., AoME 2014) whilst others were more organisation focused or about the general expected standards of healthcare professions education and thus did not detail the specific professional activities expected of a healthcare professions educator (e.g., WFME 2015). We took the decision to code such documents for their professional values only because of the difficulty in establishing the lines of activity that underlie the more generic, institution-wide standards. An example of this can be seen within the WFME *Global Standards for Quality Improvement* covering

---

How to cite this book chapter:
Browne, J., Bullock, A., Parker, S., Poletti, C., Jenkins, J., and Gallen, D. 2021. Phase 2: Analysis of Standards and Guidance Documents. *Educators of Healthcare Professionals: Agreeing a Shared Purpose*. Pp. 27–38. Cardiff, UK: Cardiff University Press. DOI: https://doi.org/10.18573/book6.c. License: CC-BY-NC-ND

Basic Medical Education (WFME 2015). The focus of the WFME standards is on their use as a tool for institutional quality improvement; thus their interest is more on what should be done rather than how it should be done and who should do it. The WFME *Global Standards* mandate that 'both teaching and student feedback must be systematically sought, analysed and responded to' (WFME 2015: 39) but what the precise role of the individual educator should be in ensuring that this takes place is not clear enough for the purposes of our study. This border of divide and overlap between the responsibilities, duties and expectations of the individual educator and the institution is part of a sector-wide conceptual challenge which we will discuss further in chapter 7.

A further six documents were also considered but later excluded from analysis upon discussion with the project team as they had either been superseded by newer standards or they were found to relate entirely to the accreditation standards of organisations rather than containing specific professional values or areas of activity.

Initial survey

As part of the survey described earlier, respondents were asked to provide details of any current standards documents that informed their practice as a healthcare professions educator. The majority of those documents listed by respondents had already been found by the research team in the literature review. However, the survey also resulted in a further ten documents being discovered that were included for analysis in this project.

In total, 48 documents were analysed in this research. For Health Education England (HEE), two relevant standards documents were identified and for the Royal Pharmaceutical Society (RPS), four relevant standards.

A full list of the 48 documents analysed in the project can be found in Appendix 1. Standards for educators in each of the professions shown in Table 1 were found and analysed except for audiologists, optometrists and orthoptists/podiatrists where we were unable to find any relevant standards for analysis. In total 38 documents were analysed for their professional values and activities and ten for their professional values only.

Analysis of Documents

Analysis of all the documents was conducted in NVivo (QSR International Pty Ltd 2018) by JB and SP. The process of analysis began with a thorough reading and re-reading of each of the standards documents at which point initial ideas about themes and codes were noted.

Initially codes were developed using the Academy of Medical Educators *Professional Standards Framework* (AoME 2014) to include all the professional values and areas of activity in this framework. The AoME Framework was chosen because it was developed through its own comprehensive and rigorous Delphi and survey processes, and because it is multidisciplinary, covering the work of educators in dentistry, medicine, veterinary science and, more recently, physician associate educators. It was also listed by many of our survey respondents as a source that they use to guide their professional practice as a healthcare professions educator.

In addition to the codes constructed from the AoME framework, we included *'The seven principles of public life'* (Committee on Standards in Public Life 1995) to ascertain whether such values were present in or had informed the standards documents. The seven principles (values) are: selflessness, integrity, objectivity, accountability, openness, honesty and leadership.

As analysis of all 48 documents proceeded, it also became clear that a number of other codes needed to be added as they were such strong themes in one or more documents. These included values/qualities such as being a role model, willingness to teach, inspiring and ethical and also activities such as engagement with stakeholders and being cost effective. A full list of codes can be found in Table 1. In total 42 codes were identified; we roughly grouped these into 21 professional values and 21 activities. The definitions we used to guide our application of codes are shown in Appendix 2.

Coding was further refined following discussions between the project team. For example, in the AoME (2014) framework teaching methods and resources are included as areas of activity twice, one in an understanding (or knows)

Table 1: List of codes used in document analysis.

Code	
Accountability	Learner wellbeing
Active learning	Learning and teaching methods, resources
Context of practice	Learning and teaching principles
Cost effectiveness	Learning needs
Development of assessment	Learning outcomes
Diversity	Management
Engagement with stakeholders	Objectivity
Equity in admissions	Openness
Ethical	Patient safety, quality of care
Evaluation of educational activity	Personal development, reflective practice in self
Evidence-based healthcare education	Person-centred
Facilitation of learning (delivery of teaching)	Professional qualification, experience

(Contd.)

Table 1: (*Contd.*)

Code	
Feedback	Purpose and methods of assessment
Governance	Quality improvement, innovation in HPE
Honesty	Quality of assessment
Inspiring	Respect for learners
Integrity	Role model
Leadership (Activity)	Safe and effective learning environment
Leadership (Value)	Selflessness
Learner progression	Teamwork, respect for colleagues, interprofessional practice
Learner reflection	Willingness to teach, enthusiasm for teaching

context and once in a uses (does) context. Upon reviewing the use of this code it became clear that many other standards documents were using these in a similar sense and thus to avoid confusion were combined into a single code called 'learning and teaching methods and resources'. Similarly, the initial codes 'assessment methods' and 'purpose of assessment' were later combined to a single code 'purpose and methods of assessment' because of the overlap between the initial coding. Finally, 'content of assessment' was merged into 'development of assessment' also because of the overlap found when coding these items. Again, this lack of clarity between 'knows', 'does' and 'believes' reflects a key faultline in how the work of the educator is understood and reflected back within standards; we discuss this further on page 98.

Findings

In this section we report separately the coding of professional values and activities. However, a table showing all coding can be found in Appendix 3.

1) Professional values/qualities

Each of the 48 documents analysed was coded for professional values and Table 2 shows the frequency of coding for each of the 21 professional values identified. Teamwork (including respect for colleagues and interprofessional practice) was the most frequently coded professional value, found in 40 of the 48 (83%) standards documents analysed. This was followed by personal development and reflective practice in self (n=38, 79%), patient safety and quality of care (n=36, 75%) and professional qualification/experience (n=36, 75%).

Table 2: Coding of professional values (number of documents=48).

Value	n
Teamwork, respect for colleagues, interprofessional practice	40
Personal development, reflective practice in self	38
Patient safety, quality of care	36
Professional qualification, experience	36
Accountability	35
Openness	34
Objectivity	32
Leadership	30
Diversity	30
Integrity	28
Learner wellbeing	28
Role Model	25
Respect for learners	23
Ethical	20
Honesty	16
Selflessness	14
Equity in admissions	11
Person-centred	11
Inspiring	10
Willingness to teach, enthusiasm for teaching	9
Context of practice	5

The values/qualities which appeared least frequently were context of practice (n=5, 10%), willingness to teach/enthusiasm for teaching (n=9, 19%) and inspiring (n=10, 20%). Overall, 12 (57%) of the 21 values appeared in more than half of the documents analysed.

2) Activities

In addition to the identification of professional values within the standards documents, we also coded 38 of the documents for the activities of a healthcare professions educator they described. As discussed above (p. 28), 10 of the documents included in the sample did not focus on individual healthcare professions educators but on educational environments and on the organisation of educational activity; and thus we took the decision to code 10 of these documents for their professional values around health professions education only.

Twenty-one professional activities were identified in the 38 standards documents, predominantly using the AoME (2014) standards as a baseline. The frequency with which each activity was coded is shown in Table 3, below. In comparison to the professional values, discussed above, overall, 16 (76%) of the 21 values appeared in more than half of the documents analysed. This suggests greater consensus as to what could be regarded as core activities than the professional values.

Table 3 shows that the most commonly coded professional activities were learning and teaching principles (n=30, 79%), learning needs (n=30, 79%) and learning and teaching methods and resources (n=29, 76%). By contrast, cost effectiveness (n=4, 11%), engagement with stakeholders (n=9, 24%) and quality of assessment (n=10, 26%) were the least commonly coded professional activities.

Table 3: Coding of professional activities (number of documents = 38).

Activity	n
Learning and teaching principles	30
Learning needs	30
Learning and teaching methods, resources	29
Learning outcomes	27
Learner Reflection	27
Purpose and methods of assessment	27
Feedback	26
Evidence based healthcare education	26
Safe and effective learning environment	25
Evaluation of educational activity	24
Governance	24
Leadership	24
Management	23
Facilitation of learning (delivery of teaching)	22
Quality improvement, innovation in HPE	21
Active learning	20
Learner progression	16
Development of assessment	16
Quality of assessment	10
Engagement with stakeholders	9
Cost effectiveness	4

3) Differences in content of professional standards documents

A total of 48 documents were analysed for this project; 10 for professional values only and 38 for professional values and shared activities. The Academy of Medical Educators' *Professional Standards for Medical, Dental and Veterinary Educators* (2014) was taken as the baseline for developing codes through which the other 47 documents were analysed because of its claim to reflect the values and activities of healthcare educators in three separate professions, but, as discussed above, a number of other codes were generated whilst analysing the sample of documents, particularly professional values. Figure 11, below, shows that the AoME (2014) framework included 30 (71%) of the 42 professional values and activities identified in this study.

Only five of the documents analysed (RPS 2015; The College of Social Work 2013; Walsh et al. 2015; World Health Organisation 2014, 2016) were found to include more of the codes than the AoME (2014) framework, suggesting that this had been a fair baseline measure to use when analysing the documents.

Summary and Conclusions

Forty-eight professional standards and guidance documents for healthcare professions educators from a range of health professions were analysed to identify core shared values and activities. The Academy of Medical Educators' *Professional Standards for Medical, Dental and Veterinary Educators* (2014) was taken as the baseline for developing codes through which the other 47 documents were analysed; this was because it was the only framework which claimed to have relevance to more than a single profession. Standards and guidance documents were found using internet search engines and on the websites of regulators/professional bodies of different healthcare professions. Responses to the initial survey resulted in a further 10 documents being identified and included in our analysis. Thirty-eight of the documents were analysed for professional values and activities, whilst a further 10 were analysed for professional values only following discussions of the organisational (rather than individual) focus of these documents amongst the project team.

Thirty codes were developed from the AoME (2014) Framework. However, a further 12 codes were added during the process of analysis that were a feature of other standards documents but not in the AoME Framework, thus bringing the total number of codes to 42 (Figure 11). Five of the documents analysed were found to have a higher number of values and areas of activity than the AoME baseline framework, with the World Health Organisation (2016) Nurse Educator Core Competencies having the most at 40. This suggests that the use of the AoME (2014) Framework, as our baseline, ws appropriate.

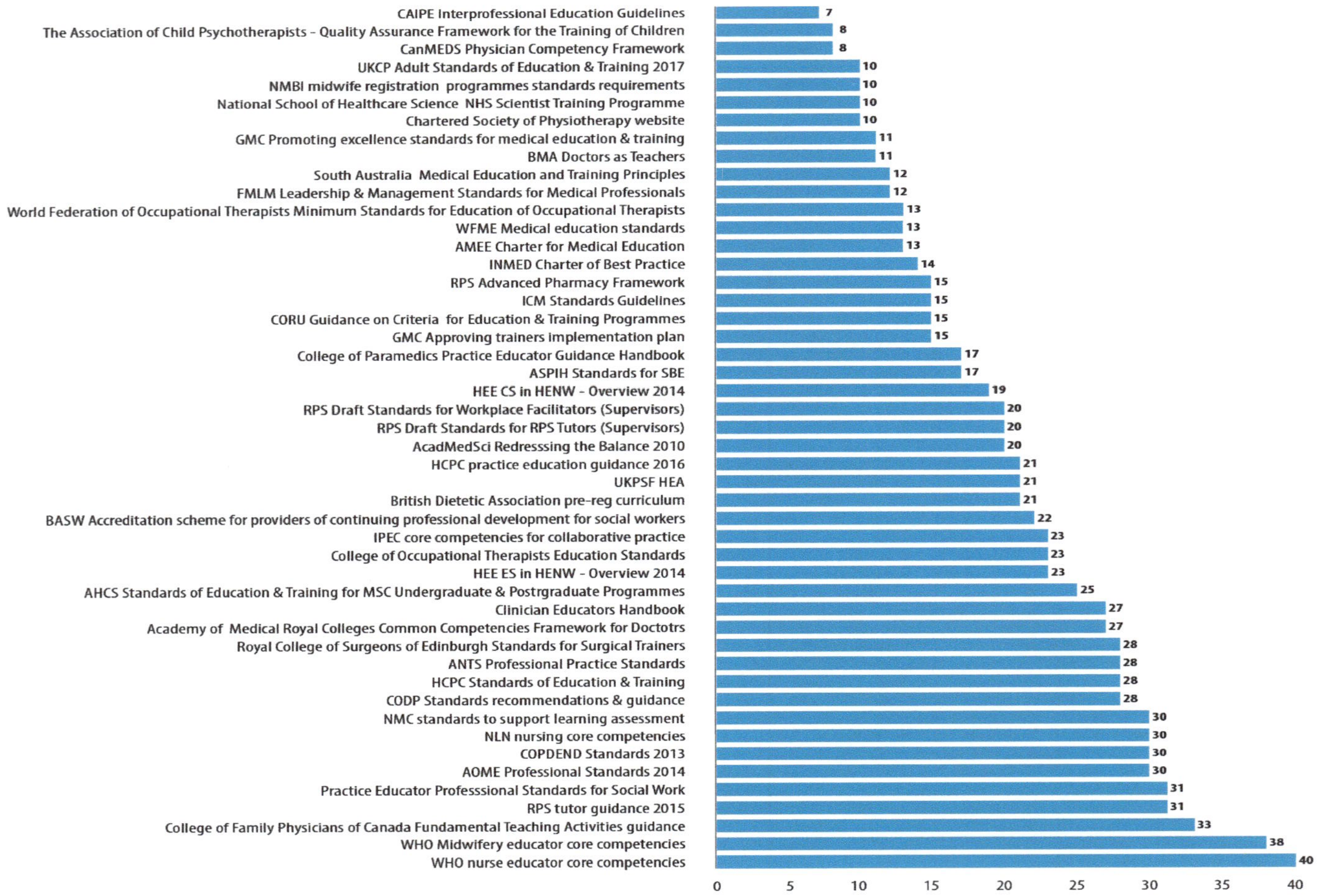

34   Educators of Healthcare Professionals

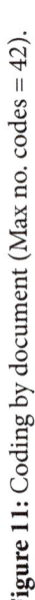

Figure 11: Coding by document (Max no. codes = 42).

Analysis of the 48 standards documents found that the most commonly occurring values were teamwork, personal development and patient safety/quality of care. However, only 12 (57%) of the 21 values were found in more than half of the documents analysed, suggesting either that there is variability in the values promoted by each of the organisations whose documents we analysed, or that the values themselves were insufficiently clearly defined in linguistic terms to be interpreted unambiguously (for example, a value such as honesty may be understood by some to include openness, ethical practice, frankness or financial probity, depending on context), or possibly both.

By contrast, there was much greater consensus when analysing the shared activities. Sixteen (76%) of the 21 values appeared in more than half of the documents analysed. This suggests greater consensus as to what could be regarded as core activities than the professional values. The most commonly occurring activities across the standards documents related to learning and teaching principles, learning needs and learning and teaching methods/resources.

This early look at the guidance supplied to educators and educational curriculum designers in a variety of professions gave us considerable optimism that common ground on basic issues could be found. Where differences were present, it was possible to trace these back as much to the structures supporting education within each profession as to any ideological views on education. Whilst detailed cross-comparisons between each profession's guidelines for good educator practice were not a part of our study design, a few sample comparisons will illustrate our point.

For example, Figure 12 shows how NVivo software (QSR International Pty Ltd 2018), used to code the COPDEND *Professional Standards for Dental Educators* (Committee of Postgraduate Dental Deans and Directors 2013) and the Nursing and Midwifery Council (NMC) *Standards to Support Learning and Assessment in Practice* (2008), compares the two side by side. The first thing to note is the enormous central overlap between the two documents. Of all the values and activity codes generated, fully 28 are common to each document. It is the differences that are interesting: the COPDEND standards require educators, in addition to the 28 areas shared with the NMC standards, to demonstrate openness, selflessness, a commitment to diversity and an understanding of admissions processes. While the NMC standards look for an ability to deliver intended learning outcomes, a commitment to quality of assessment and learner wellbeing and an understanding of the context of practice and student progression (all essential in teaching environments where progress relies on the satisfactory completion of a portfolio of competences), they notably require their teachers to possess professional licensure – something that was not found in many other guidelines where interprofessional learning and wider teaching teams were the norm.

A similar comparison (Figure 13) between the Academy of Medical Sciences' *Redressing the Balance* guidelines (Academy of Medical Sciences 2010)

36 Educators of Healthcare Professionals

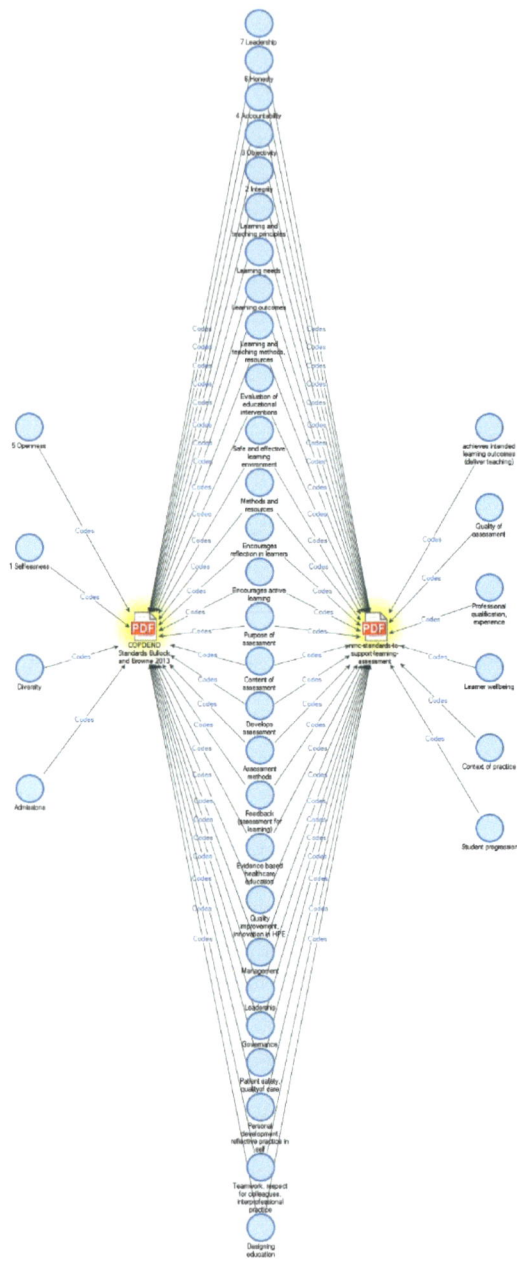

Figure 12: Coding comparison between the COPDEND *Professional Standards for Dental Educators* (Committee of Postgraduate Dental Deans and Directors 2013) and the Nursing and Midwifery *Council Standards to Support Learning and Assessment in Practice* (2008).

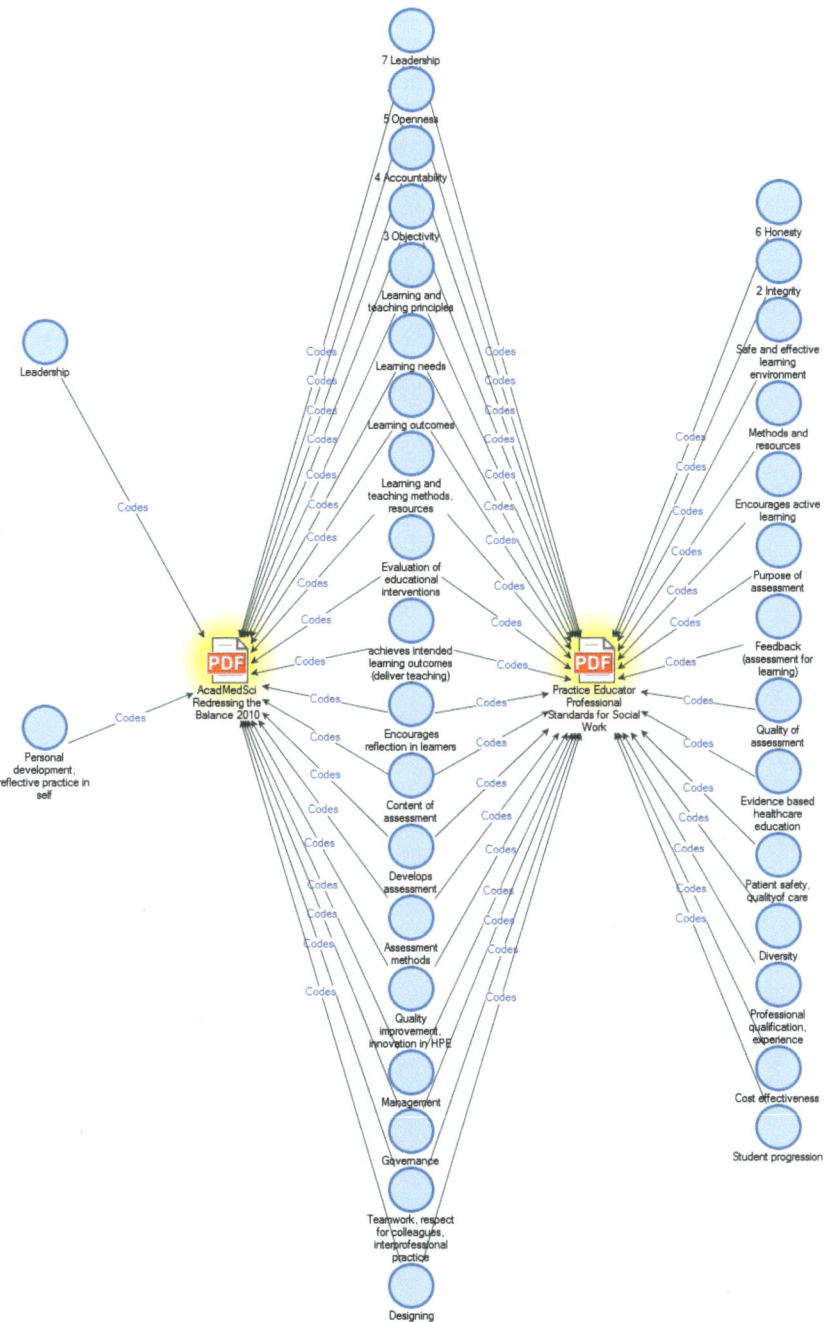

Figure 13: Coding comparison between *Redressing the Balance* (Academy of Medical Sciences 2010) and the College of Social Work *Practice Educator Professional Standards for Social Work* (2013).

and the College of Social Work's *Practice Educator Professional Standards for Social Work* (College of Social Work 2013) shows, once again, that 19 values and activities are shared. In this case, however, while the Academy of Medical Sciences guidelines require a further two elements not shared by the College of Social Work standards – leadership and a commitment to personal development – the College of Social Work requires a further 14 values and activities. Several of these additional themes reflect the fact that social work teaching, unlike science teaching, may take place with clients and service users present alongside learners, and also that the work of the social work educator is ultimately to prepare learners for work with clients and service users – hence the addition of such items as safe and effective learning environment, patient safety and evidence-based healthcare.

CHAPTER 4

Phase 3: The Nominal Group

The Nominal Group Process

Nominal group technique is a consensus method that is used to explore a topic, assess the extent of agreement and resolve disagreement (Delbecq et al. 1986). The 'expert' participants gathered together for a day's meeting. Following an outline of the day and an overview of the study, as a warm-up activity, the participants were invited to discuss what they thought were key issues for their profession currently. The rest of the day was divided into two main parts which followed a similar process: the first focused on values and the second on activities. Each part began with a presentation of the outcomes of the document analysis. The items were discussed and clarified resulting in some items being combined and new items added. This agreed list was then voted on. For the voting, each participant had six voting cards (two cards with three points; two cards with two points; and two cards with one point). Each participant then privately assigned their six voting cards to six of the items that they judged most important. The facilitator collated the results and the voting outcomes were then displayed to the group and discussed. Following further amendments, the group then voted a second time. The second vote allowed participants to modify their choices in the light of the feedback from Round 1. The results were then tabulated and fed back to the group.

The Participants

A nominal group is made up of experts, in this case carefully selected senior individuals who had held a significant role as a healthcare educator (teacher, support or regulator) in the United Kingdom or Ireland. Our participants

---

How to cite this book chapter:
Browne, J., Bullock, A., Parker, S., Poletti, C., Jenkins, J., and Gallen, D. 2021. Phase 3: The Nominal Group. *Educators of Healthcare Professionals: Agreeing a Shared Purpose*. Pp. 39–48. Cardiff, UK: Cardiff University Press. DOI: https://doi.org/10.18573/book6.d. License: CC-BY-NC-ND

were identified from the work in the earlier phases of the study (survey and documents analysis) and suggestions from the advisory group. Our main aim was to get wide coverage of (a) professional groups (b) geographical representativeness from all four nations within the British Isles plus Ireland and (c) individuals with a broad range of experience at undergraduate, postgraduate and continuing professional education.

Participation was voluntary. Eight senior HCEs took part in the meeting, which was held on Friday 14th September 2018 at Friends House in London.

Results

Current issues for educators

In nominal groups, the discussion that accompanies the voting process may sometimes be more significant than the voting itself. From our analysis of the discussions, we identified four cross-cutting themes that arose throughout the day.

Looking to the future

This theme was mainly about innovation and technology in education and the need to keep pace with change. For example, one expert commented on 'the rapid pace of innovation and change' and the need to 'make sure that what we teach is fit for the future health service'. This was echoed by others who made reference to the 'changing labour force', 'changing student demography'. A strong case was made by one participant who emphasised the importance of ensuring that education was up-to-date with technological innovation: 'the way that people learn now is very different, and we have to completely change the way we educate'.

Policies and funding

Reference was made to policy development and the implications this has for educational funding. One participant observed the 'increasing divergence on how healthcare educations are seen and how they are funded'. Comment was made about the need to fund continuing education of educators and researchers: 'without educators, people in the job will simply reproduce things as they already are'. Uncertainty about future funding was linked to Brexit, staff shortages and cuts to education funding. It was also noted that Ireland, as the only English-speaking country in the European Union, was expecting increased pressure for registration and the recognition of qualifications.

Patients

Patients, and their place in education, were mentioned by several participants. For example, one commented on what they thought was a current 'lack of involvement of patients or service users in health education'. This was linked by another participant to changing expectations of service users.

Interprofessional learning

Interprofessional education was a recurrent theme throughout the day. At the outset, one individual commented on what they perceived as the 'big problem of lack of communication across professions'.

Values

Initial items and discussion

The first question that the group addressed was: how central to the educator role are the following personal qualities and values? Table 4 shows the list of values initially presented to the group and the second column indicates if the item was grouped with another item or changed.

From the discussion, 'professionalism' emerged as an additional, broad value and the group agreed to subsume three items within this: ethical conduct, honesty and integrity. Before deciding on the term 'professionalism', the group considered calling the value 'trustworthy professionalism' or 'professional behaviour' but settled on 'professionalism'.

The group noted that the list did not include 'effective communication' and how that might relate to openness and role modelling. There was some discussion that communicating was better related to activities rather than values but a new item 'communication' was included in Round 1 voting.

A number of other values were brought under the 'fairness' umbrella: context of practice, diversity, equity in admissions and respect for others. The decision to include context of practice within 'fairness' was driven by the fact that 'context of practice' was the code which captured statements such as the need for educators to 'ensure that learners attending a practice placement receive high-quality practice education whatever the context or setting' (Health and Care Professions Council (HCPC) 2017). That is to say it was invariably linked to consistency of education quality, an essential element if all students are to develop to their maximum potential.

'Leadership' attracted considerable discussion. It was seen as connected to role modelling and inspiring others. Although difficult to define, the group agreed to leave it in for Round 1 voting.

Table 4: Initial values and modifications.

#	Value	Change
#1	Accountability	
#2	Context of practice	Subsumed under fairness
#3	Diversity	Subsumed under fairness
#4	Equity in admissions	Subsumed under fairness
#5	Ethical conduct	Subsumed under professionalism (new item)
#6	Honesty	Subsumed under professionalism (new item)
#7	Inspiring	Clarified as including an ability to challenge ideas
#8	Integrity	Subsumed under professionalism (new item)
#9	Leadership	Problematic to define and may be part of 'inspire and challenge'
#10	Learner wellbeing	Modified to: concern for learner wellbeing
#11	Objectivity	Removed
#12	Openness	Subsumed under communication (new item)
#13	Patient safety, quality of care	
#14	Personal development, reflective practice in self	Modified to: personal development, reflective practice in self and others
#15	Person-centred	
#16	Professional qualification, experience	Uncertain meaning: personal development? or teaching with level of competence?
#17	Respect for learners	Modified to: respect for others. Then subsumed under fairness
#18	Role model	
#19	Selflessness	
#20	Teamwork, respect for colleagues, interprofessional practice	
#21	Willingness to teach, enthusiasm for teaching	Subsumed under inspiring and challenging

Amended items and first round voting

Further modifications were made:

- Personal development, reflective practice in self and others: modified to personal <u>and professional</u> development, reflective practice in self.

Table 5: First round voting.

Value	n votes
Professionalism	20
Inspiring and challenging	18
Communication (openness)	15
Personal development, reflective practice in self and others	10
Role model	9
Fairness	7
Patient safety, quality of care	6
Person-centred	6
Concern for learner wellbeing	3
Teamwork, respect for colleagues, interprofessional practice	3
Professional qualification, experience	2
Accountability	1
Leadership	0
Selflessness	0

- Teamwork, respect for colleagues, interprofessional practice. In discussion, respect for colleagues was seen as part of professionalism and/or a part of fairness. Teamwork was seen as discrete from interprofessional practice. Interprofessional learning was emphasised over interprofessional practice. The item was changed to 'values interprofessional learning'. And 'respect for others' was added to 'fairness'.
- Professional qualification, experience: removed. In discussion the participants noted that qualification and experience are not values and that not all educators (for example non-clinical educators, expert patients or educators from certain healthcare groups) have professional qualifications in healthcare. Still fewer have professional qualifications in education.

Second round voting

Prior to Round 2 voting, it was decided to exclude 'professionalism' from the list as consensus had been achieved after Round 1. The results of Round 2 voting are displayed in Table 6.

'Communication' moved up to second place. 'Inspiring and challenging' maintained prominence and 'values interprofessional learning' attracted significant votes.

Table 6: Second round voting.

Value	n votes
Professionalism [consensus after R1 so removed from R2 voting]	/
Communication	24
Inspiring and challenging	19
Values interprofessional learning	13
Fairness and respect for others	10
Personal and professional development, reflective practice in self and others	7
Role model	7
Patient safety, quality of care	4
Person-centred	4
Concern for learner wellbeing	3
Accountability	0
Leadership	0
Selflessness	0

Activities

Initial items and discussion

The second question that the group addressed was: how central to the educator role is the knowledge of, making use of or development of the following activities? Table 7 shows the list of activities initially presented to the group and the second column indicates if the item was grouped with another item or modified.

The group quickly decided to amalgamate 'learning and teaching methods, resources', 'learning and teaching principles', 'learning needs' into a more general activity they named 'efficient and effective learning and teaching'. This activity was then used as the umbrella for 'active learning', 'cost effectiveness', 'facilitation of learning' and 'management'. They decided to keep 'learning outcomes' separate and clarify this by adding the word 'identify' at the start. They did not reach agreement on whether 'safe and effective learning environment' should be a part of 'efficient and effective learning and teaching', so they kept them separate for Round 1 voting.

The group discussed the relationship between learning, teaching and assessment. They noted that 'quality of assessment' and 'development of assessment' should go together and are linked to 'learning outcomes'. Following discussion about feedback and assessment, they suggested that feedback should remain as a separate item but the other items discussed should be part of a new item they

Table 7: Initial activities list and modifications.

#	Educational Activity	Change
#1	Active learning	Subsumed under efficient and effective learning and teaching (new item)
#2	Cost effectiveness	Subsumed under efficient and effective learning and teaching (new item)
#3	Development of assessment	Subsumed under assessment fit for purpose (new item)
#4	Engagement with stakeholders	Modified to: engagement with others
#5	Evaluation of educational activity	
#6	Evidence based healthcare education	Modified to: evidence informed healthcare education
#7	Facilitation of learning (delivery of teaching)	Subsumed under efficient and effective learning and teaching (new item)
#8	Feedback	Modified to: feedback, progression and reflection
#9	Governance	Subsumed under quality assurance, improvement and enhancement
#10	Leadership	
#11	Learner progression	Subsumed under feedback
#12	Learner reflection	Subsumed under feedback
#13	Learning and teaching methods, resources	Subsumed under efficient and effective learning and teaching (new item)
#14	Learning and teaching principles	Subsumed under efficient and effective learning and teaching (new item)
#15	Learning needs	Subsumed under efficient and effective learning and teaching (new item)
#16	Learning outcomes	Modified to: identify appropriate learning outcomes
#17	Management	Subsumed under efficient and effective learning and teaching (new item)
#18	Purpose and methods of assessment methods	Subsumed under assessment fit for purpose (new item)
#19	Quality improvement, innovation in HPE	Modified to: quality assurance, improvement and enhancement. The 'innovation' aspect added as a new item plus another new item technology to enhance learning
#20	Quality of assessment	Subsumed under assessment fit for purpose (new item)
#21	Safe and effective learning environment	

called 'assessment fit for purpose'. Also 'learner progression' and 'learner reflection' became part of 'feedback'.

The item 'quality improvement, innovation in HPE' was separated and modified to 'quality assurance, improvement and enhancement' (to which the item 'governance' was added) and the 'innovation' aspect developed as a new item. After discussion about innovation, a further new item was added which they called 'technology to enhance learning'.

Amended items and first round voting

Further modifications were made:

- Engagement with others: modified to 'engagement with others (stakeholders)'. Participants felt that this linked more effectively to interprofessional education, and that engagement with others would be implicit in 'efficient and effective learning and teaching'.
- There was concern that the activities should look to the future and that 'innovation' fails as a term to capture the idea of 'preparedness for futures' (the idea of learning to learn, to innovate and adapt in response to the changing healthcare and education environments). This was added as a new item for Round 2.

Second round voting

Prior to Round 2 voting, it was decided to exclude 'effective and efficient teaching and learning' from the list as consensus had been achieved after Round 1.

Table 8: First round voting.

Activity	n votes
Effective and efficient learning and teaching	24
Evaluation of educational activity	13
Feedback, progression and reflection	9
Innovation	9
Technology to enhance learning	9
Engagement with others	7
Assessment fit for purpose	7
Quality assurance, improvement and enhancement	6
Evidence informed healthcare education	5
Safe and effective learning environment	5
Identify appropriate learning outcomes	2
Leadership	0

Table 9: Second round voting.

Activity	n votes
Effective and efficient learning and teaching	/
Feedback, progression and reflection	17
Engagement with others	17
Preparedness for futures	12
Evaluation of educational activity	11
Innovation	11
Technology to enhance learning	8
Quality assurance, improvement and enhancement	8
Evidence informed healthcare education	5
Assessment fit for purpose	3
Safe and effective learning environment	3
Identify appropriate learning outcomes	1
Leadership	0

The results of Round 2 voting are displayed in Table 9. 'Feedback' and 'engagement with others' moved up towards the top of the table. The new item, 'preparedness for futures' attached significant votes and 'innovation' held its place. The distance between 'assessment fit for purpose' and 'evaluation of educational activity' widened as evaluation took precedence.

Final Remarks

The experts were invited to offer some final comments. Their parting messages included:

- The view that it needs to be acknowledged more widely that the term 'educator' is very broad and includes learning in the workplace and in different disciplines. However, they wanted the view to be recorded that the educator is a person; and that if they are good in their role, the context (setting or discipline) is immaterial.
- They wanted a more coherent recognition from regulators and within education that educating others is part of professional practice.
- They felt strongly that skills in interprofessional and teamworking were too easily taken for granted – like educational skills – and needed to be more explicitly fostered and developed.
- They were concerned that rank-and-file educators would find it difficult to appreciate the relevance of standards to their practice and felt that the benefits would need to be clearly stated and linked to a reward system that

would encourage engagement with any standards framework that might be developed in the future.
- Education needs to be valued as highly as service delivery.

The final voting patterns of the nominal group were interesting, but as is often the case in nominal groups, it was the discussion and reconciliation of conflicting perspectives that generated the richest data to inform the project. We were aware that the participants in the nominal group were very senior and represented leaders and policy makers within the healthcare professions rather than classroom or clinical teachers, which would give their perspectives a particular bias. This turned out to be the case; it was apparent from the results that these individuals were used to 'big picture' thinking, to leading and co-ordinating large teams, to future gazing and to sustainability and succession planning in healthcare. It will be seen from our findings that they tended to favour activities and values associated with these aspects of healthcare education planning in their responses.

CHAPTER 5

Phase 4: Workshop

Methods

At a meeting of the International Network for Health Workforce Education (INHWE) in Dublin (9–10 January 2019) a workshop was held at which two of the authors (JJ and JB), acting as facilitators, presented the background and context of the study, together with the methods and headline results of the first two phases. They also announced the start of the Delphi study with the intention of recruiting from the audience, which was a mixed group of around 90 international health professions educators, mainly from Europe but also from Canada, the United States and a number of African countries.

Following a short presentation on the background to the study and the purpose of the workshop, most of the session was devoted to an activity aimed at eliciting the views of the audience on whether any organising principles could be applied to the 42 codes used in the document analysis (see Tables 2 and 3).

The delegates were asked to sit at tables in groups of up to 10 and were given felt pens, flipchart paper and sheets of repositionable labels pre-printed with the 42 codes. They were then given the following instructions:

(1) All groups should read the labels and sort them into sub-groups. Give each sub-group a title explaining the organising principle.

(2) While doing this, decide:

Are there any items missing? Make a new label.
Are there any items that need amalgamating? Position them together.
Are there any items that are not needed at all? Put these to one side.
Are there any items that need renaming? Rename them.

After just over half an hour the flip-chart worksheets were collected, together with any unused labels.

How to cite this book chapter:
Browne, J., Bullock, A., Parker, S., Poletti, C., Jenkins, J., and Gallen, D. 2021. Phase 4: Workshop. *Educators of Healthcare Professionals: Agreeing a Shared Purpose.* Pp. 49–70. Cardiff, UK: Cardiff University Press. DOI: https://doi.org/10.18573/book6.e. License: CC-BY-NC-ND

Results

The delegates who took part in the exercise were divided into nine groups. Each group produced a poster.

Before reporting on each group's organisation of the items, we begin by outlining our general observations on the results of the activity.

Values

- Not all groups distinguished values from areas of activity. Those who did, did not necessarily identify the same values that had previously been identified in the analysis of documents. Some groups included items that had previously been identified as activities.
- When giving a title to the 'values' group, numerous synonyms were offered, including: professionalism, attributes and qualities.
- Some items – such as 'diversity' – were perceived as a personal value while others viewed it as an institutional value, responsibility or activity.
- There was some doubt about how to document the 'unmeasurable' personal qualities that some educators possess. Some qualities are in the eye of the beholder and are impossible to define or assess objectively. This could make it difficult to require that educators should possess qualities such as inspiring, role model and openness.

Of the seven groups that grouped values, Table 9 shows both commonality and diversity. In terms of commonality, at least five of the seven groups included: respect for colleagues, honesty, openness, integrity and ethical conduct. Group 1's response was unlike others: of the six items identified by Group 1 as 'values', three of these were not included by any other group. Their items labelled 'behaviours' were more akin to those labelled 'values' by other groups. In contrast, there was much commonality between Groups 5 and 6 and between Groups 7 and 8.

Figure 14 provides a visual overview of the most employed labels under the grouping 'values'/ 'principles'. It is possible to distinguish the group of 'core' labels that have been used by the majority of groups, these are: honesty, openness, ethical conduct, integrity, respect for colleagues, selflessness, willingness/ enthusiasm. Table 10 shows the distribution of items and degree of consensus between groups.

Some labels are only mentioned once, such as: active learning, encourages reflection in learners, equity in admission, evidence-based education, interprofessional practice, leadership, learner wellbeing, professionalism, quality improvement, reflective practice in self (self-reflection), role model use of resources.

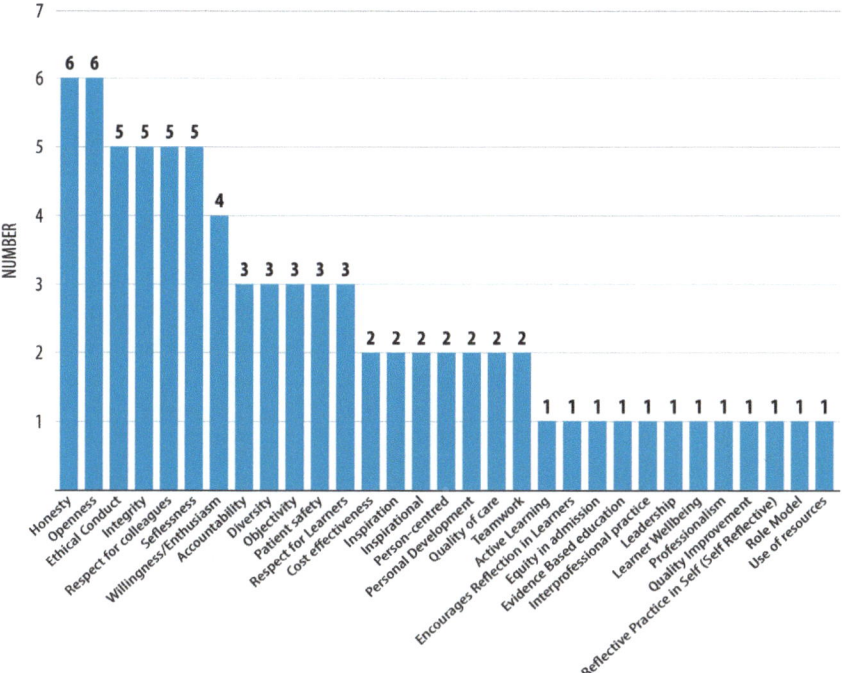

Figure 14: Overview of frequency of distribution of values and principles.

Table 10: Items grouped as values.

Values	Group 1	Group 3	Group 5	Group 6	Group 7	Group 8	Group 9	Tot
Interprofessional practice	x							1
Patient safety	x				x	x		3
Quality Improvement	x							1
Quality of care	x				x			2
Cost effectiveness	x	x						2
Evidence Based education	x							1
Equity in admission		x						1
Respect for colleagues		x	x	x	+team-work		+team-work	5
Selflessness		x	x		x	x	x	5

(Contd.)

Table 10: *(Contd.)*

Values	Group 1	Group 3	Group 5	Group 6	Group 7	Group 8	Group 9	Tot
Honesty		x	x	x	x	x	+professionalism	6
Accountability		x	x			x		3
Diversity		x				x	x	3
Use of resources		x						1
Inspirational		x			x	x	x	4
Openness		x	x	x	x	x	x	6
Integrity			x	x	x	x	x	5
Respect for Learners			x	x			x	3
Ethical Conduct			x	x	x	x	x	5
Willingness/ Enthusiasm				x	x	x	x	4
Objectivity				x		x	x	3
Person-centred					x	x		2
Learner Wellbeing					x			1
Personal Development						x	x	2
Active Learning						x		1
Reflective Practice in Self						x		1
Encourages Reflection in Learners							x	1
Role Model							x	1
Leadership							x	1

Activities

- Activities were also subdivided in ways that suggested that it was not clear to delegates what the appropriate level of responsibility should be: activities were ascribed as personal or as a function of the programme, its governance or related to institutional support.
- No one used the rather simplistic categorisation 'delivery of teaching' even though this is in common use in some professions' educator guidance. This was unexpected as, although the participants were all healthcare educators of some seniority, and while in some professions 'facilitation of learning' is in more common usage, 'delivery of teaching' is still current. Group 5 was the only one that included teaching methods as a heading.

Some used the pre-printed labels but crossed them out. Others wrote new terms on the labels.

Sub-groups

The groups followed different organising principles to create sub-groups using the labels, and in large part they do not coincide. However, general traits common to the majority of the sub-grouping rationales can be identified:

1. The distinction between values (or principles) and activities.
2. The distinction between individual attributes and attributes at the level of organisation/institution.
3. Some groups included something similar to cause–effect relationships by connecting labels with directions and arrows, or by defining certain labels as outcomes of other (e.g., Group 4 added the label 'faculty service collaboration' as a sort of 'end point' signalled by arrows; Group 5 specified a list of labels as being part of learning outcomes. Similarly, Group 6 included a whole list under the label 'outcomes').
4. Group 2 suggested the amalgamation of 'learning and teaching methods and principles'; but the large majority of the groups used the two labels together, as if they were part of the same concept.

We provide further detail on each of the group's response to the activity in turn.

Group 1

Group 1 divided the labels into core goals and three main sub-groups (behaviours, attributes and structures and methods) and included a list of ungrouped labels (see Figure 15 and Table 11). The group introduced new labels under the sub-group 'core values': these were Evidence-Based Practice (EBP), Continuing Professional Development (CPD), Communication (with the addition of: 'conflict?') and Role Clarity. They defined leadership as conflict management.

Table 11: How Group 1 ordered the items.

Behaviours	Attributes	Structures and methods	Core goals values
Accountability	*Ethical conduct/Respect for colleague	Assessment development (+AKA design)	Interprofessional practice
Honesty	*Integrity/Respect for learners	Assessment quality	Patient safety
Reflective practice in self	*Leadership (Conflict management)	Assessment purpose/methods	Quality Improvement
Objectivity	Professional qualification/ experience	Governance	Quality of care
Willingness/enthusiasm	Personal development (LLL)	*Person-centred learning outcomes	Cost effectiveness
*Ethical conduct/ Respect for colleague	Learner wellbeing	Learner progression	Evidence Based education
*Integrity/Respect for learners	Active learning	Learning and teaching principles	
Openness	Teamwork	Safe/effective learning environment	+EBP
Selflessness	Diversity (+inclusive, 2 levels surface and deep)	Context of practice	+CPD
*Person-centred learning outcomes	Role model	Use of resources (+availability of resources)	+Communication (conflict?)
*Leadership (Conflict management)	Inspiration	Learning and teaching methods/ Facilitation of learning	+Role clarity
	+Operations Management	Evaluation of education	
		Stakeholder engagement	
		Learning needs (+?)	
		Feedback + Method	
		Encourages reflection in learners	
		+Practice academic partnership	
		+Infrastructure	

* Is used when labels appear under different sub-groups.
+ Is used to indicate new labels added by the groups.

Phase 4: Workshop 55

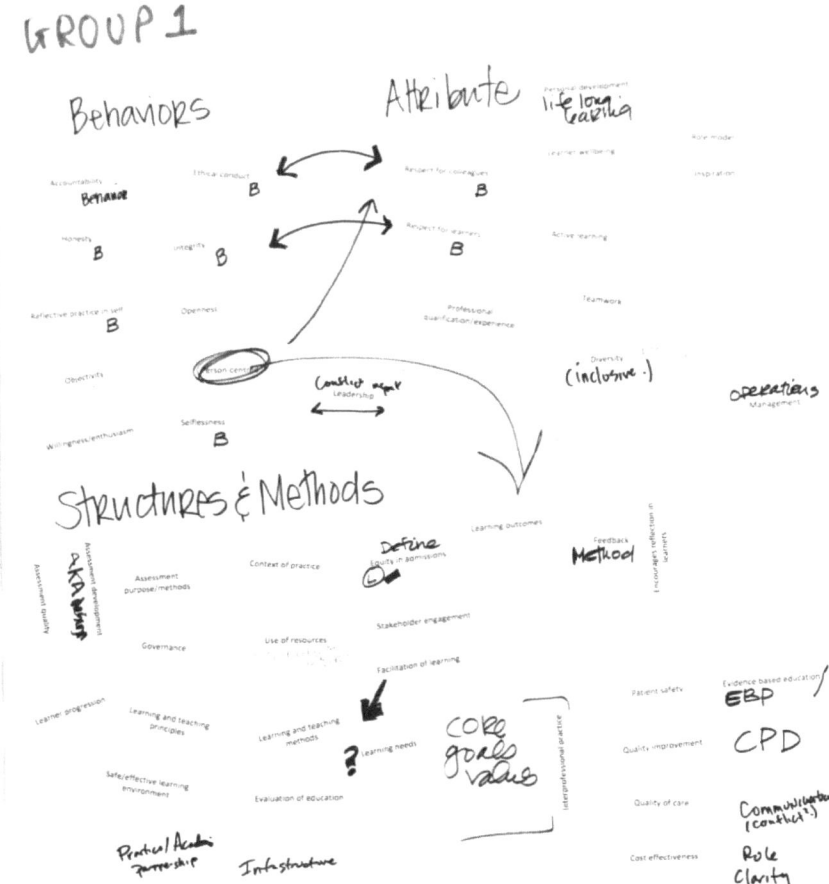

Figure 15: Group 1 worksheet.

Group 2

Group 2 adopted a slightly different approach from all other groups, by presenting a summary explaining the rationale behind the sub-group division, based on the identification of overarching themes. They did not order the items into a table (Figure 16). They explained:

Issues such as the following are **overarching themes:**

1. **Ethical issues** (integrity, honesty, ethical conduct, respect for colleagues, learners, person centred, etc.).

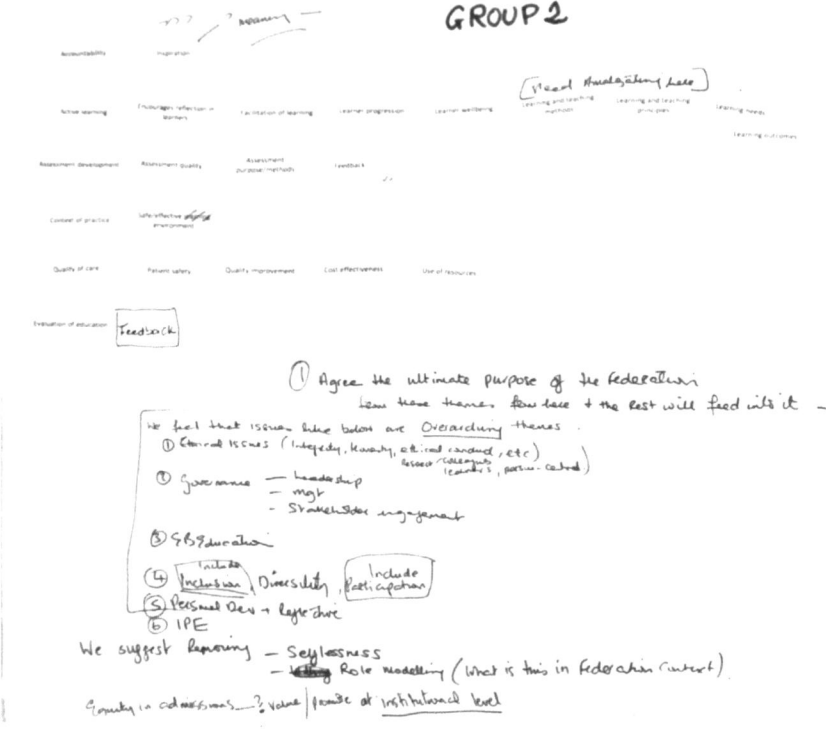

Figure 16: Group 2 worksheet.

2. **Governance** (leadership, management, stakeholder engagement).
3. **Evidence-based education.**
4. **Include** inclusion, diversity, include participation.
5. **Personal development** and reflection.
6. **IPE.**

We suggest **removing** selflessness, role modelling, learning from 'safe/effective learning environment'. Equity in admission: which is a value to be promoted at the institutional level.

In other comments they asked for clarification of 'inspiration' and suggested the amalgamation of 'learning and teaching methods and principles'.

Group 3

Group 3 separated values from activities (Figure 17 and Table 12). They introduced the activity 'mentoring' and the sub-group 'peer review'. They created and crossed the label: 'educator wellbeing'.

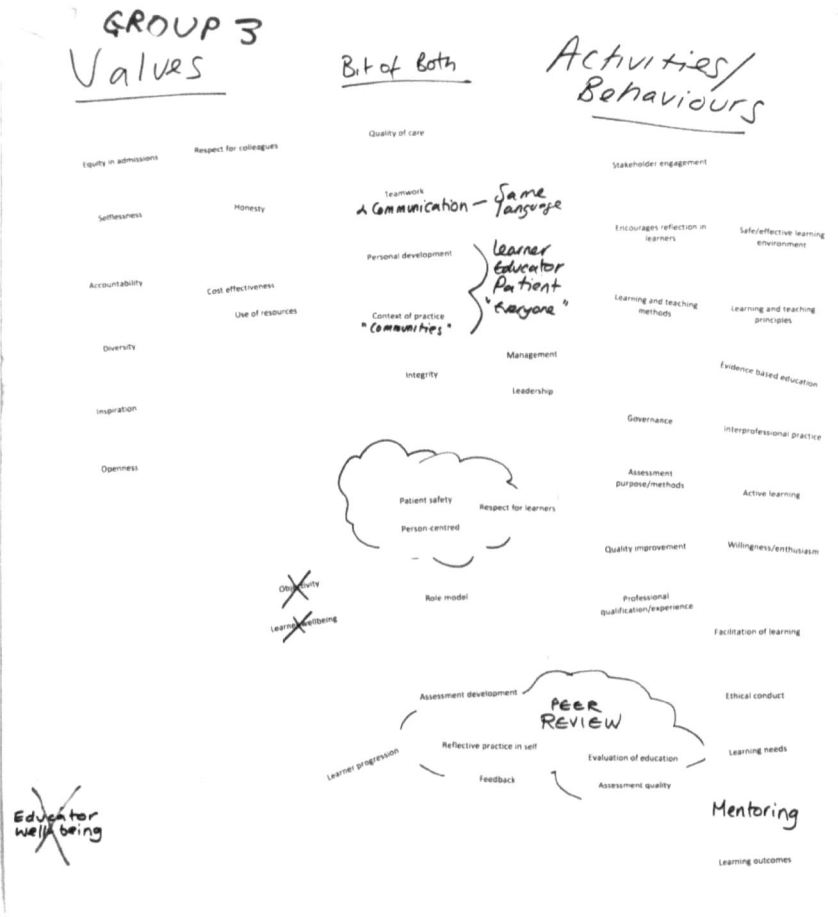

Figure 17: Group 3 worksheet.

Table 12: How Group 3 ordered the items.

Values	Activities/behaviours	Bit of both	Peer review	Not used/crossed out or added
Equity in admission Respect for colleagues Selflessness Honesty Accountability Cost effectiveness Diversity Use of resources Inspiration Openness	Stakeholder engagement Encourages reflection in learners Learning and teaching methods Governance Assessment purpose/method Quality improvement Professional qualification/experience Safe/effective learning environment Learning and teaching principles Evidence based education Interprofessional practice Active learning Willingness/enthusiasm Facilitation of learning Ethical conduct Learning needs Learning outcomes +Mentoring	Quality of care Teamwork + Communication Personal development Context of practice + 'Communities' = learner, educator, patient, everyone Integrity Management Leadership [Patient safety, respect for learners, person-centred] Role model	Assessment development, Learner progression, Reflective practice in self, Feedback, Evaluation of education, Assessment quality	Objectivity Learner well-being +Educator well-being

* Is used when labels appear under different sub-groups.
+ Is used to indicate new labels added by the groups.

Group 4

Group 4 introduced a special category for management/organisational support (an institutional level) and distinguished this from educational processes in general. They include a sub-group specifically about quality, with the addition of the item 'quality metrics'. They do not use the label 'values' but do distinguish 'personal attributes'. They included a new label; 'faculty service collaboration', as outcome of the other sub-groups (Figure 18 and Table 13).

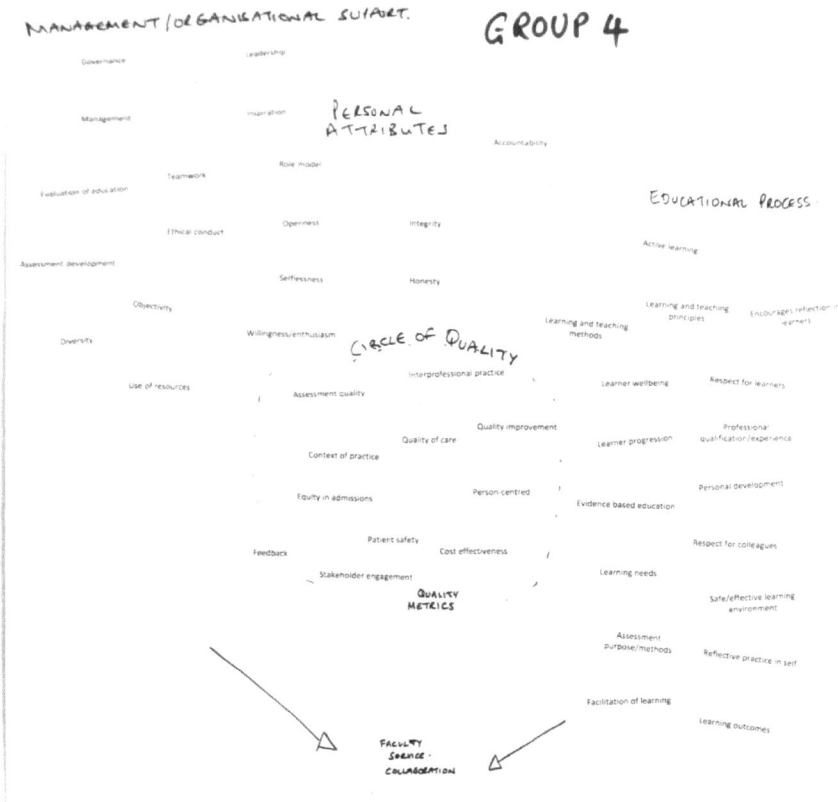

Figure 18: Group 4 worksheet.

Table 13: How Group 4 ordered the items.

Management / organisational support	Unclear, in between the two	Personal attributes	Circle of quality	Educational process
Governance	Objectivity	Leadership	Assessment quality	Active Learning
Management	Use of Resources	Inspiration	Context of practice	Learning and Teaching Methods/Principles
Evaluation of education	Teamwork	Role model	Equity in admissions	Learner Wellbeing
Assessment development	Ethical conduct	Openness	Feedback	Learner Progression
Diversity		Selflessness	Patient safety	Evidence Based Education
		Willingness/ Enthusiasm	Stakeholder engagement	Learning Needs
		Integrity	Cost effectiveness	Assessment Purpose/Method
		Honesty	Person-centred	Facilitation of Learning
		Accountability	Quality of care	Encourage Reflection in Learners
			Quality improvement	Respect for Learners
			Interprofessional practice	Professional Qualification/Experience
			+Quality metrics	Personal Development
				Respect for Colleagues
				Sage/Effective Learning Environment
				Reflective Practice in Self
				Learning Outcomes
faculty service collaboration (as result)				

* Is used when labels appear under different sub-groups.
+ Is used to indicate new labels added by the groups.

Group 5

Group 5 distinguished values as part of professionalism and identified four other sub-groups (plus one of not used labels) (Figure 19 and Table 14).

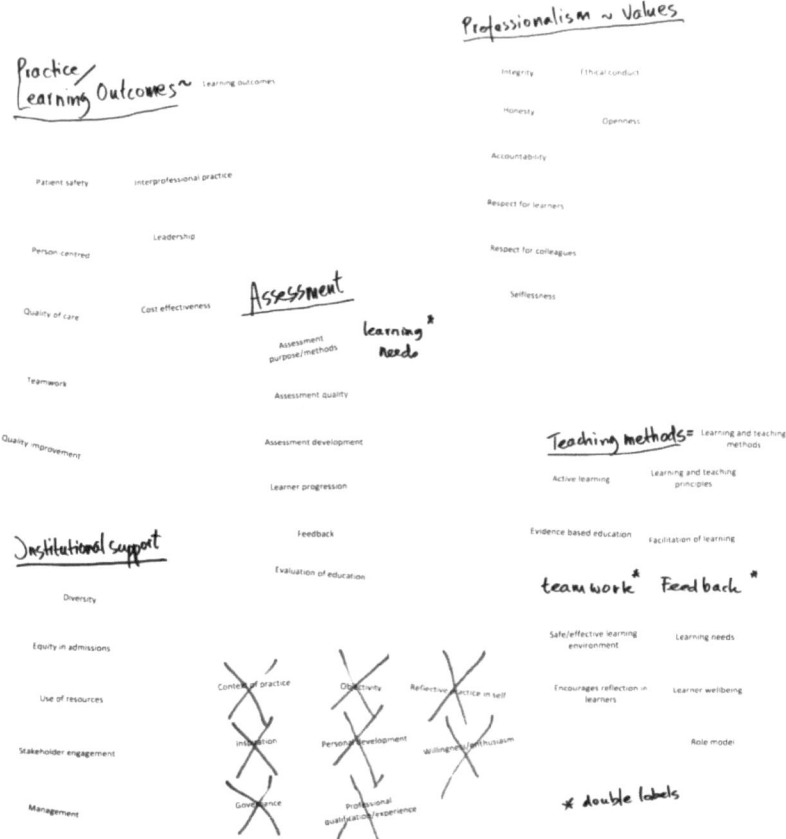

Figure 19: Group 5 worksheet.

Table 14: How Group 5 ordered the items.

Practice/Learning Outcomes	Institutional Support	Assessment	Professionalism Values	Teaching Methods / Learning and Teaching Methods	Not Used
Patient Safety, Person-centred Quality Of Care, Teamwork, Quality Improvement, Interprofessional Practice, Leadership, Cost Effectiveness	Diversity, Equity in Admission, Use of Resources, Stakeholder-Engagement, Management	Assessment Purpose/Method, Assessment Quality, Assessment Development, Learner Progression, Feedback, Evaluation Of Education, *Learning Needs	Integrity Honesty Accountability Respect for Learners Respect for Colleagues Selflessness Ethical Conduct Openness	Active Learning Learning And Teaching Principles EBE Facilitation of Learning *Teamwork *Feedback Safe/Effective Environment Learning Needs Encourage Reflections in Learners Learner Wellbeing Role model	Context Of Practice Objectivity Reflective Practice In Self Inspiration Personal Development Willingness/Enthusiasm Governance Professional Qualification/Experience

* Is used when labels appear under different sub-groups.
\+ Is used to indicate new labels added by the groups.

Group 6

Group 6 separated values from other sub-groups (which were labelled learning competences, process of care/learning and outcomes (Figure 20 and Table 15). Process of care/learning was sub-divided into 'Learning process elements' and 'context'. Also in this case, personal competencies are distinguished from the general learning process.

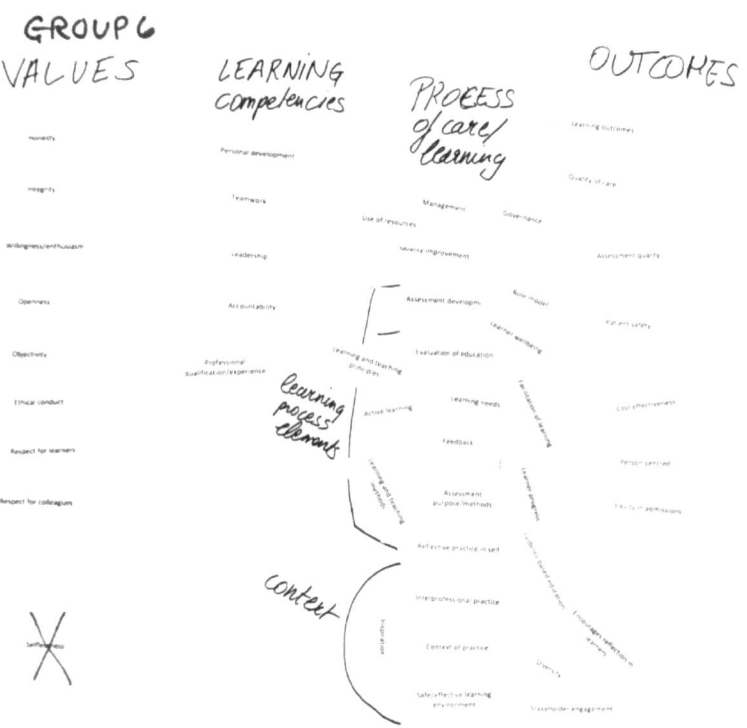

Figure 20: Group 6 worksheet.

Table 15: How Group 6 ordered the items.

Values	Learning Competencies	Process of Care/Learning	Outcomes	Not Used
Honesty	Personal Development	Management	Learning Outcomes	Selflessness
Integrity	Teamwork	Governance	Quality Of Care	
Willingness/Enthusiasm	Leadership	Use of Resources	Assessment Quality	
Openness	Accountability	Quality Improvement	Patient Safety	
Objectivity	Professional Qualification/	Learning Process Elements:	Cost Effectiveness	
Ethical Conduct	Experience	Assessment Development	Person-Centred	
Respect For Learners		Role Model	Equity in Admission	
Respect For Colleagues		Learner Wellbeing		
		Evaluation Of Education		
		Learning and Teaching Principles/Methods		
		Active Learning		
		Learning Needs		
		Feedback		
		Assessment Purpose/Methods		
		Facilitation of Learning		
		Learner Progression		
		Reflective Practice In Self		
		Context:		
		Interprofessional Practice		
		Context Of Practice		
		Inspiration		
		Safe/Effective Learning Environment		
		Evidence Based Education		
		Encourage Reflection		
		Diversity		
		Stakeholder Engagement		

* *Is used when labels appear under different sub-groups.*
+ *Is used to indicate new labels added by the groups.*

Group 7

Group 7 separated those things that they considered to be the role of the institution, or the institution through the agency of the educator (i.e. programme governance) from the more clearly individual aspects (i.e. activity, educator attributes and values) (Figure 21 and Table 16).

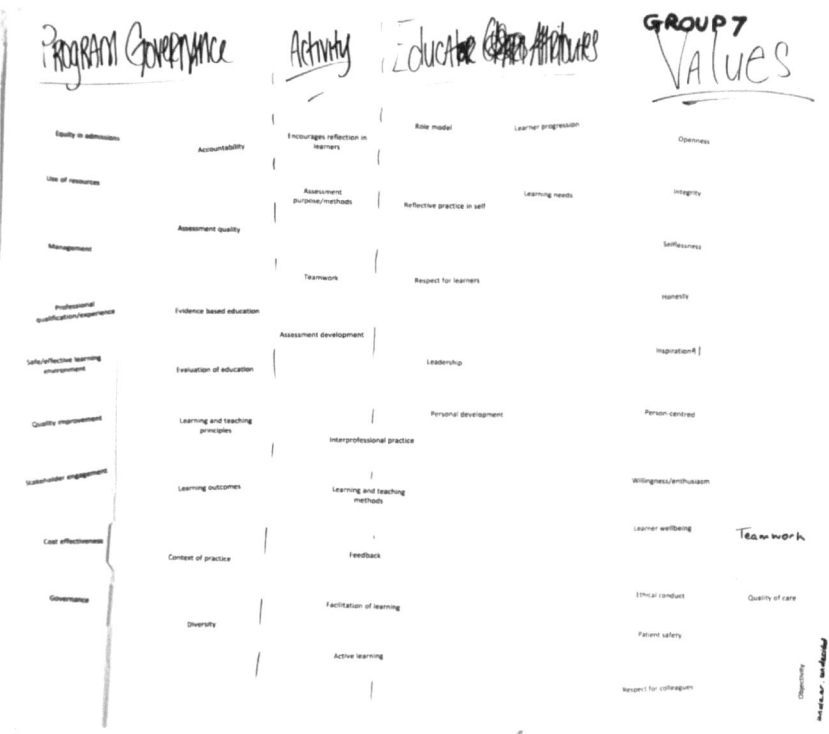

Figure 21: Group 7 worksheet.

Table 16: How Group 7 ordered the items.

Programme Governance	Activity	Educator Attributes	Values
Equity in Admissions	Encourages Reflection in Learners	Role Model	Openness
Use of Resources	Assessment Purpose/Methods	Reflective Practice In Self	Integrity
Management	Teamwork	Respect for Learners	Selflessness
Professional Qualification/Experience	Assessment Development	Leadership	Honesty
Safe/Effective Learning Environment		Personal Development	Inspiration(al)
Quality Improvement		Learner Progression	Person-centred
Stakeholder Engagement		Learning Needs	Willingness/Enthusiasm
Cost Effectiveness			Learner Wellbeing
Governance			Ethical Conduct
Accountability			Patient Safety
Assessment Quality			Respect for Colleagues
Evidence Based Education			+Teamwork
Evaluation of Education			Quality Of Care
Learning and Teaching Principles			Objectivity (Undecided/Unclear)
Learning Outcomes			
Context of Practice			
Diversity			

* Is used when labels appear under different sub-groups.

+ Is used to indicate new labels added by the groups.

Group 8

Group 8 separated the general principles from principles/values and qualities that belong to the individual level (Figure 22 and Table 17).

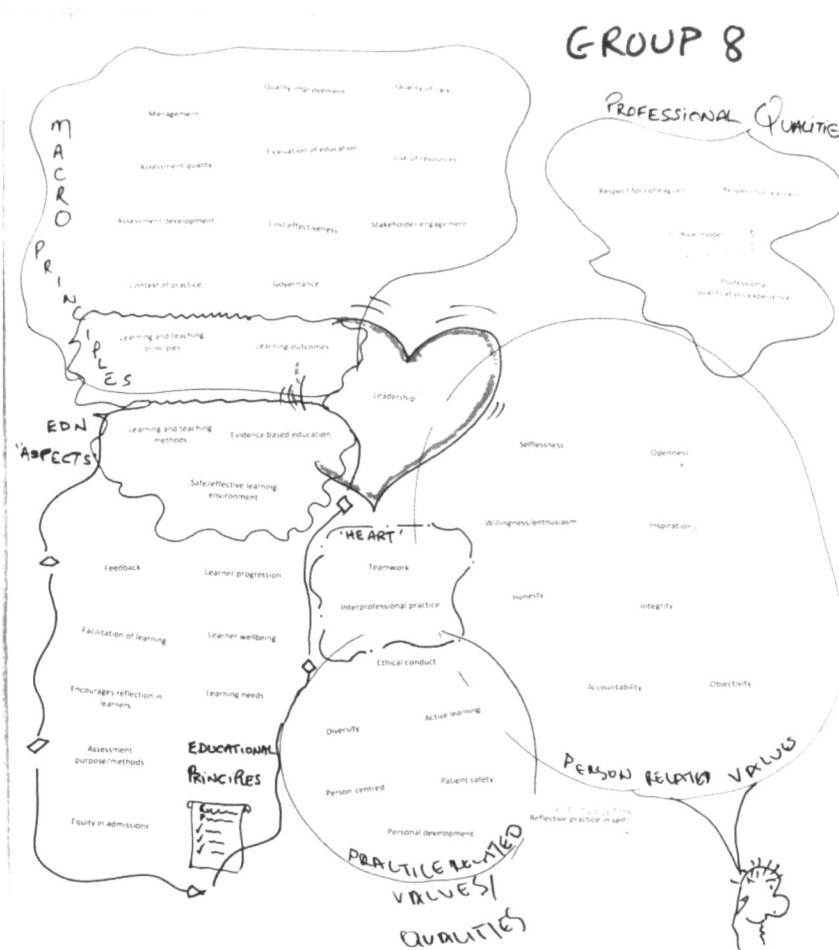

Figure 22: Group 8 worksheet.

Table 17: How Group 8 ordered the items.

Macro Principles	Educational Principles	Heart	Practice Related Values/Qualities	Person Related Values	Professional Qualities
Management	**EDN Aspects**	Leadership	Ethical Conduct	Selflessness	Respect for Colleagues
Assessment Quality	Learning And Teaching Methods	Teamwork, Interprofessional Practice	Diversity	Willingness/ Enthusiasm	Respect for Learners
Assessment Development	Evidence Based Education		Person-centred	Honesty	Professional Qualification/ Experience
Context of Practice	Safe/Effective Learning Environment		Personal Development	Openness	Role Model (Seems?)
Quality Improvement			Active Learning	Inspiration(+al)	
Evaluation of Education			Patient Safety	Integrity	
Cost Effectiveness	Feedback		Reflective Practice In Self (Self Reflective)	Accountability	
Governance	Facilitation of Learning			Objectivity	
Quality of Care	Encourages Reflection In Learners				
Use of Resources	Assessment Purpose/ Methods				
Stakeholder Engagement	Equity in Admission				
Learning and Teaching Principles	Learner Progression				
Learning Outcomes	Learner Wellbeing				
	Learning Needs				

* Is used when labels appear under different sub-groups.
+ Is used to indicate new labels added by the groups.

Phase 4: Workshop   69

Group 9

This group separated values from activities that they grouped under the headings 'foundation', 'patient experience' and 'extra' (Figure 23 and Table 18).

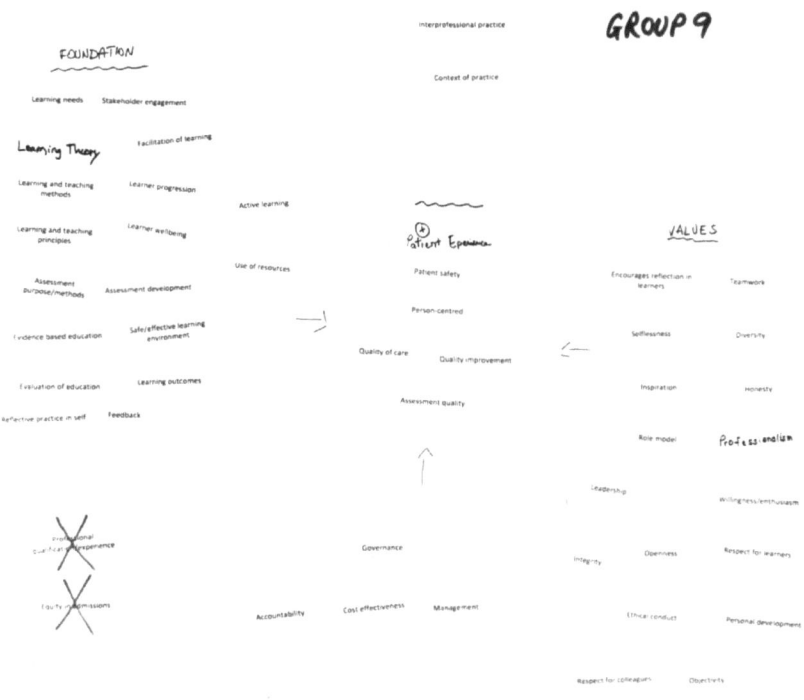

Figure 23: Group 9 worksheet.

Table 18: How Group 9 ordered the items.

Foundation	Values	Patient Experience	Extra	Not Used
Learning Needs	Encourages Reflection in Learners	Patient Safety	Governance	Professional Qualification/Experience
+Learning Theory	Selflessness	Person-centred	Accountability	Equity in Admission
Learning and Teaching Methods/Principles	Inspiration	Quality Of Care	Cost Effectiveness	
Assessment Purpose/Methods	Role Model	Quality Improvement	Management	
Evidence Based Education	Leadership	Assessment Quality	Interprofessional Practice	
Evaluation of Education	Integrity		Context of Practice	
Reflective Practice In Self	Openness			
Stakeholder Engagement	Ethical Conduct			
Facilitation of Learning	Respect For Colleagues			
Learner Progression	Teamwork			
Learner Wellbeing	Diversity			
Assessment Development	Honesty			
Safe/Effective Learning Environment	+Professionalism			
Learning Outcomes	Willingness/Enthusiasm			
Feedback	Respect for Learners			
Active Learning	Personal Development			
Use of Resources	Objectivity			

* Is used when labels appear under different sub-groups.
+ Is used to indicate new labels added by the groups.

CHAPTER 6

Phase 5: The Delphi Study

The Delphi Process

Delphi is a consensus method in which participants respond to two or three rounds of the survey. At the second round, participants are invited to reassess their answers based on the anonymous aggregate results of the first round and respond again only to the items which did not reach consensus. This process may continue for a further, third round, as required (de Villiers et al. 2005). This was not necessary in our study.

Consensus criteria

In order to identify the items that achieved consensus, we applied the following criteria:

- At least 80% of participants rated the item as essential/desirable or committed/highly committed (i.e., > 80% giving a rating of 3 or 4).
- AND the mean rating > 3.4.
- AND the standard deviation < 1.0.

We note that there is no agreed recommendation for setting the level of consensus (Powell 2003). We are aware too of the debate about the acceptability of using means and standard deviations with Likert rating scales (Carifio & Perla 2008; Norman 2010). Following others (for example Diamond et al. 2014; Hand 2006), we judged that the mean and standard deviation were helpful in revealing the tendency or degree of the opinions.

How to cite this book chapter:
Browne, J., Bullock, A., Parker, S., Poletti, C., Jenkins, J., and Gallen, D. 2021. Phase 5: The Delphi Study. *Educators of Healthcare Professionals: Agreeing a Shared Purpose.* Pp. 71–93. Cardiff, UK: Cardiff University Press. DOI: https://doi.org/10.18573/book6.f. License: CC-BY-NC-ND

Overview of the Rounds

In the first round, participants were asked to rate on a 4-point scale[1] their commitment, as healthcare educators, to nine values and to judge 33 areas of educational activity as essential, desirable, optional or not necessary. The values and activities were derived from the 42 codes used in the document analysis, modified in the light of the nominal group and the INHWE workshop. The INHWE activity revealed some ambiguity in terms of the distinction between values and activities; for example, some respondents felt that interprofessional education (IPE) is an activity, not a value. The nominal group was helpful in condensing the values. Those in the nominal group also condensed the activities; however, for the purpose of the Delphi we determined that it would be more helpful to disaggregate the activities to allow a wider breadth of choice. We identified nine values and 33 activities for the Delphi. These indicative activities were loosely arranged into five areas: preparation, teaching and supporting learning, learner progression, working in teams and enhancing quality. Additionally, participants were given an opportunity to comment on aspects of the items or suggest additional items.

As a result of Round 1, eight out of the nine values and 22 out of 33 the activities achieved consensus. In Round 2, participants were invited to consider the 12 items which did not achieve consensus at Round 1. For each, they were given details of the results and invited to submit a second rating. Three of the 12 items then achieved consensus at Round 2.

The Participants

Recruitment was primarily by social media. For the purpose of recruitment, tweets containing a link to an online survey were sent out between 14 and 28 January 2019. Both the Academy of Medical Educators and CUREMEDE publicised the link to the survey through their accounts (@medicaleducator and @curemede) which gave access to their followers (10,700 and 1,272 respectively), most of whom have an interest in healthcare education. Various accounts retweeted the link, giving an engagement rate in the tens of thousands. Hashtags and tagging specific accounts were used to promote the survey to other healthcare education organisations during the first week; as responses to the survey were received, the second week's tweets were tailored to attract the attention of the smaller, less-represented professions: e.g., in an attempt to recruit audiologists we used #hearing @BAAudiology @audiologyonline @BSAudiology1; similar efforts were made to attract the interest of other professional healthcare education organisations.

Participants were also recruited via email. The email contact lists included participants that had already been involved in the Nominal Group as well as members of relevant bodies (such as COPDEND).

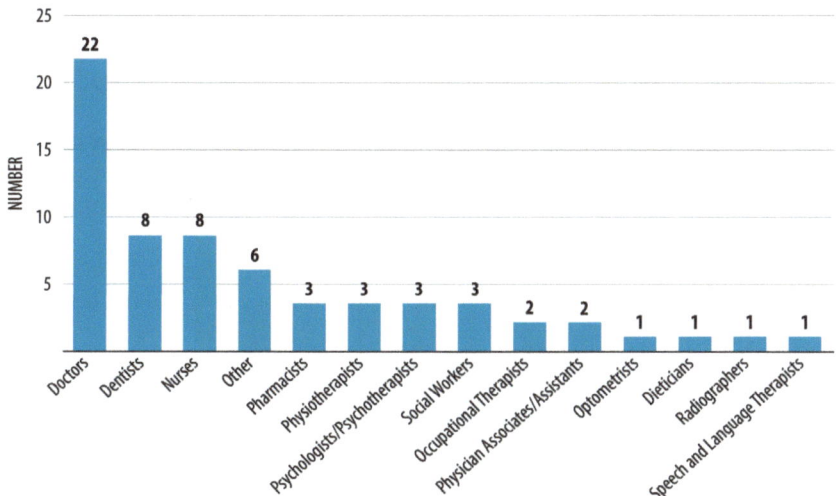

Figure 24: Affiliations of Round 1 Delphi group participants.

Round 1 of the survey was taken by 37 participants[2] (who declared themselves to be actively involved in the provision of healthcare education or healthcare standards and/or a healthcare trainee/student or practitioner in the United Kingdom or Ireland.

Respondents identified the health or social care professional groups to which they belonged, educated or regulated. They could select more than one of: doctors, dentists, nurses, pharmacists, physiotherapists, psychologists/psychotherapists, social workers, occupational therapists, physician assistants, optometrists, dieticians, radiographers, speech and language therapists, biomedical scientists, audiologists, orthoptists/podiatrists/chiropodists and other.

Respondents from Round 1 covered a broad spectrum of health and social care professional groups (see Figure 24). The majority of participants (n=22) relate to the professional group of doctors, followed by dentists (n=8), nurses (n=8) and members of 'other' groups specifically ODPs, healthcare scientists (medical physics, physiological sciences and life sciences in healthcare), midwives, multiprofessional educators, dental care professionals, undergraduate medical students.

The only groups with no representation are audiologists, biomedical scientists and orthoptists.

Round 1 Results

In the first part of Round 1, participants were invited to express their level of commitment to nine core values for healthcare educators.

The values presented were:

1. **Ethical conduct**: Working within appropriate governance, legal frameworks and relevant professional codes of conduct.
2. **Upholding patient wellbeing and safety**: Performing the educator role with due consideration for the wellbeing, dignity and safety of patients; balancing the needs of high quality healthcare delivery with the needs of high quality healthcare education.
3. **(High) Quality in education**: Developing, promoting, advancing and providing high quality healthcare education; inspiring and supporting learners
4. **Respect for learners**: Considering the needs of both individuals and groups of learners; acting with consideration for the emotional, physical and psychological wellbeing of learners.
5. **Fairness:** Ensuring, promoting and respecting equality of opportunity and diversity in all aspects of the healthcare educator role.
6. **Respect for colleagues**: Responding appropriately to feedback; teamwork, collaboration; supporting colleagues in their personal and professional development.
7. **Accountability**: Transparency and openness in educator practice, including revealing competing interests.
8. **Personal development as an educator**: Maintaining and enhancing personal practice through analysis, reflection and feedback on the educator role; using evidence to inform educator practice.
9. **Interprofessional education**: Supporting inter-, trans- and multi-professional education; learning with, from and about other healthcare professionals to improve collaborative care; actively working to address barriers to collaboration.

Values: Round 1 Results

According to our consensus criteria, eight out of the nine values presented in the list achieved consensus. The distribution of replies was skewed in favour of a commitment towards all the values in the list. The majority of participants' choices lean towards 'committed' or 'highly committed' (see Figure 25).

Interprofessional education was the only value that did not reach the threshold for consensus in Round 1, since its mean was <3.4 (see Table 19). It is the only item that any respondent rated 'uncommitted'. For this reason, the item was included in the second round of the Delphi.

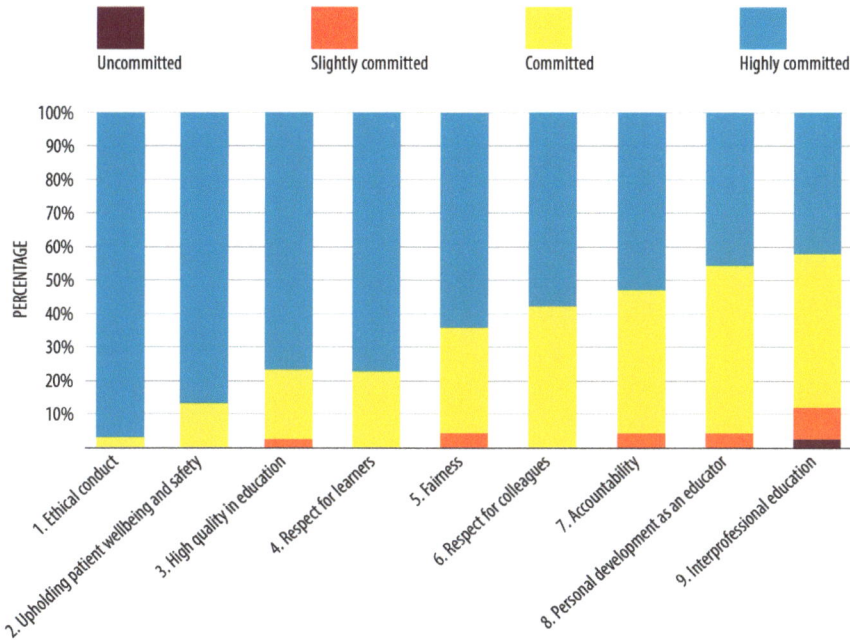

Figure 25: Delphi group Round 1 rating of values (full axis labels are given in Table 19).

Table 19: Round 1 results for values, ordered by mean.

Value	Combined Committed /Highly committed	Mean	SD	Count
Ethical conduct	100.0%	3.97	0.16	37
Upholding patient wellbeing and safety	100.0%	3.89	0.31	37
Respect for learners	100.0%	3.78	0.41	37
(High) Quality in education	97.3%	3.76	0.49	37
Fairness	94.6%	3.59	0.59	37
Respect for colleagues	100.0%	3.59	0.49	37
Accountability	94.6%	3.51	0.60	37
Personal development as an educator	94.6%	3.43	0.59	37
Interprofessional education	86.5%	3.27	0.76	37

Table 20: Round 1 comments about the values.

Comment	Number of times mentioned
All are important	9
Clarity needed on accountability	2
Hard to separate some	1
Comprehensive	1
Additional items: • self-care • professional inclusivity? breadth of professional vision (instead of IPE) • excellence in clinical practice • respect for patients • political advocacy for learners	1 1 1 1 1

Comments about the list of values

Fourteen respondents added a comment. Most commonly, respondents indicated that they thought that all the values were important. Some participants reported 'accountability' as too ambiguous: one remarked that it was not clear if the value referred to students or the profession; another questioned whether accountability was a value, suggesting rather that it was 'mainly related to governance of the institution'. A summary of the comments is presented in Table 20.

The activities: Round 1 results

The second part of Round 1 concerned activities. Participants rated the following groups of activities: preparation for teaching and learning, teaching and supporting learning, learner progression, working in teams, enhancing quality.

According to the consensus criteria described above, out of 33 single activities, 22 achieved consensus. In general, participants' rating of the different items in the lists of activities were skewed towards positive positions (i.e., ratings of 3 and 4). However, compared to the responses for values, the items rated under activities were more dispersed.

Activities – Preparation for teaching and learning

In this group, the list of activities comprised:

1. Aligns planned activities with the intended learning outcomes.
2. Identifies the learning needs of students.

3. Defines learning outcomes and subject content.
4. Understands the (changing) context of learning environment (e.g., regulation, workforce).
5. Understands how principles of teaching and learning are applied to the preparation of teaching.
6. Demonstrates an awareness of a range of learning and teaching methods.
7. Makes effective use of resources (human, financial resources and learning technologies).

According to the consensus criteria all seven activities achieved consensus, and for this reason were not included in the second round of the survey. These activities were rated mostly as either 'desirable' or 'essential' (i.e., frequency above 80%); the mean was above 3.4 and standard deviation below 1.0 (see Table 21 and Figure 26).

Within these results, 'defines learning outcomes and subject content' was the more 'divisive' among the activities presented and included one participant who considered it 'not necessary' and another only 'optional'. This is reflected in the comments (see Table 22 and related discussion).

Comments about preparation of teaching and learning

Eleven respondents added a comment. Most commonly, respondents indicated that they thought that all activities were important. As highlighted above

Table 21: Round 1 activities results for preparation for teaching and learning, ordered by mean.

Activities	Desirable/ Essential	Mean	SD	Count
Aligns planned activities with the intended learning outcomes	100.0%	3.78	0.41	37
Identifies the learning needs of students	100.0%	3.76	0.43	37
Understands the (changing) context of learning environment (e.g. regulation, workforce)	100.0%	3.65	0.53	37
Understands how principles of teaching and learning are applied to the preparation of teaching	94.6%	3.64	0.48	36
Defines learning outcomes and subject content	97.3%	3.62	0.67	37
Demonstrates an awareness of a range of learning and teaching methods	94.6%	3.57	0.59	37
Makes effective use of resources (human, financial resources and learning technologies)	94.6%	3.43	0.59	37

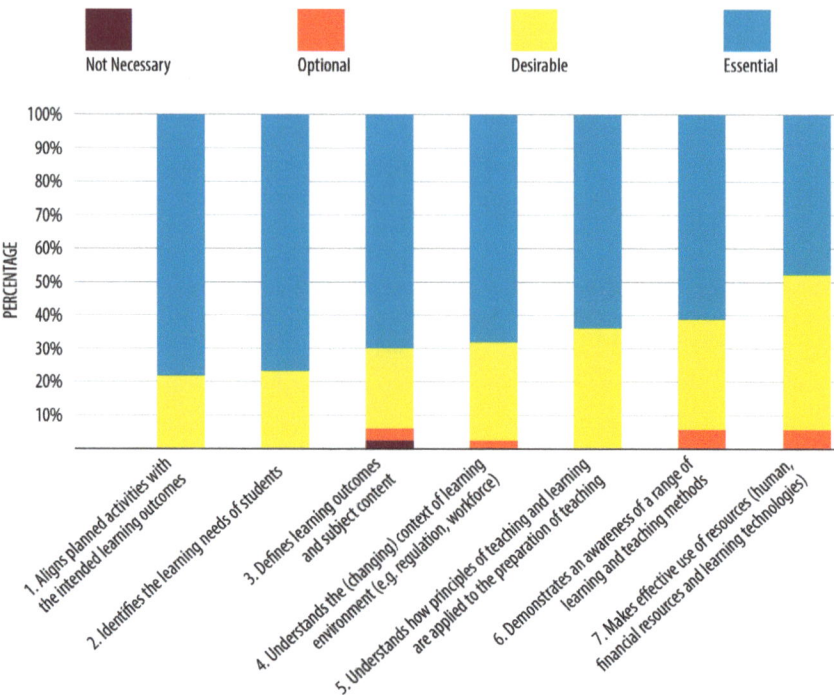

Figure 26: Delphi group Round 1 rating of Activities 1 – Preparation for teaching and learning (full axis labels are given in Table 21).

(Figure 26), two participants rated 'Defines learning outcomes and subject content' as 'not necessary' or 'optional'. Two comments offer some explanation for such ratings: 'you can be a very effective educator delivering LOs and content defined by others', 'Sometimes an effective educator does not need to define learning outcomes and subject content in advance – a more free-flowing approach can result in valuable unexpected outcomes'. Another comment suggested that defining learning outcomes depends on the amount of resources available. The importance of resources was also referred to (one comment) in relation to the introduction of new technologies: 'it would be good to be able to do this but access to resources/tools to do this is limited and also in healthcare we can have different groups at each teaching session so it is not possible to do this'. Another comment stressed how some of the activities related to the preparation of teaching and learning depend on the nature of the specific roles occupied, as 'a Dean will definitely need to know about regulators and workforce, but a new lecturer probably not'. A summary of the comments is reported in Table 22.

Table 22: Round 1 comments on preparation of teaching and learning.

Comment	Number of times mentioned
All are important	4
Defining LOs is not necessary for an educator	2
Depends on resources	3
Depends on role	1
Additional items: • Learning science should be included in 'Understands how principles of teaching and learning are applied to the preparation of teaching'	1

Activities – Teaching and supporting learning

In this group, the list comprised:

1. Balances the needs of learners with the need to provide safe patient care.
2. Establishes a safe and effective learning environment.
3. Applies principles of adult learning to their teaching practices.
4. Uses a range of educational methods and technologies to help students achieve intended learning outcomes.
5. Manages educational resources in a cost-effective manner.

According to the consensus criteria, three of these five activities achieved consensus. The activities 'Uses a range of educational methods and technologies to help students achieve intended learning outcomes' and 'Manages educational resources in a cost-effective manner' did not reach the threshold for consensus since their means were lower than 3.4 (see Figure 27 and Table 23).

Comments about teaching and supporting learning

Seven respondents added a comment. The majority of comments stressed how activities such as cost management and establishing a safe learning environment should not be considered among the responsibilities of educators (see Table 24). This was explained as either because: 'establishing a safe and effective learning environment is not always in the gift of the educator...', or because '... the Head of dept, should have to worry about the financial aspects'. Another respondent commented that cost management is not important as it is 'not directly pertinent to the quality of the education delivered'. Another comment stressed how establishing a safe learning environment does not depend on the

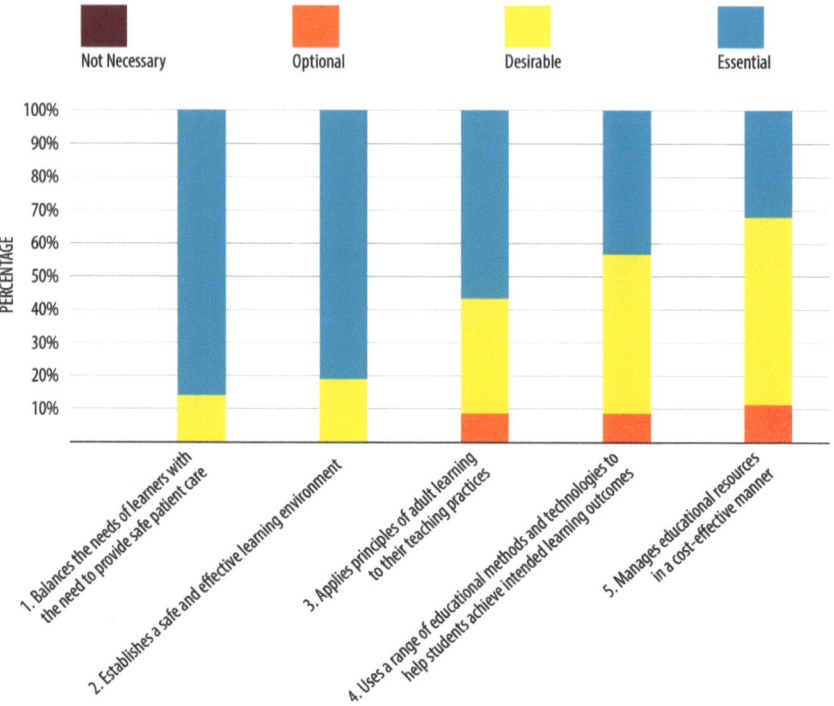

Figure 27: Delphi group Round 1 rating of Activities 1 – Teaching and supporting learning (full axis labels are given in Table 23).

Table 23: Round 1 activities results for teaching and supporting learning, ordered by mean.

Activities	Desirable/ Essential	Mean	SD	Count
Balances the needs of learners with the need to provide safe patient care	100.0%	3.86	0.34	37
Establishes a safe and effective learning environment	100.0%	3.81	0.39	37
Applies principles of adult learning to their teaching practices	91.9%	3.49	0.64	37
Uses a range of educational methods and technologies to help students achieve intended learning outcomes	91.9%	3.35	0.62	37
Manages educational resources in a cost-effective manner	89.2%	3.22	0.62	37

Table 24: Round 1 comments on teaching and supporting learning.

Comment	Number of times mentioned
Not an educator responsibility	3 (2 concerning safe learning environment, 1 cost management)
Cost management is important	1
Cost management is *not* important	1
Adult learning is *not* the only theory	1
Reference to adult learning is *not* necessary	1

educator but rather on the type of teaching: 'the balance of safe patient care becomes much more important with clinical teaching for me'. A summary of comments is presented in Table 24.

Activities – Learner progression

In this group, the list comprised:

1. Provides learner-centred and timely feedback to learners.
2. Selects appropriate methods to assess learners' progress.
3. Links assessment to learning outcomes.
4. Supports learner engagement in reflective practice.
5. Understands a range of methods to assess learners' progress.
6. Evaluates and improves assessments.
7. Contributes to the construction of assessments.

According to the consensus criteria, five out of the seven activities achieved consensus. 'Evaluates and improves assessments' and 'Contributes to the construction of assessments' did not reach the threshold, since their mean values were lower than 3.4. In the case of 'Contributes to the construction of assessments' the responses also did not reach the 80% threshold for desirable and essential combined (see Figure 28 and Table 25).

Comments about learner progression

Seven respondents added a comment. In this case, three comments stressed how 'evaluates and improves assessments' or 'contributes to the construction of assessments' should not be considered among the responsibilities of educators, either because 'a very effective educator could be delivering assessments defined by others' or because 'assessment is one of the areas which needs a lot of work

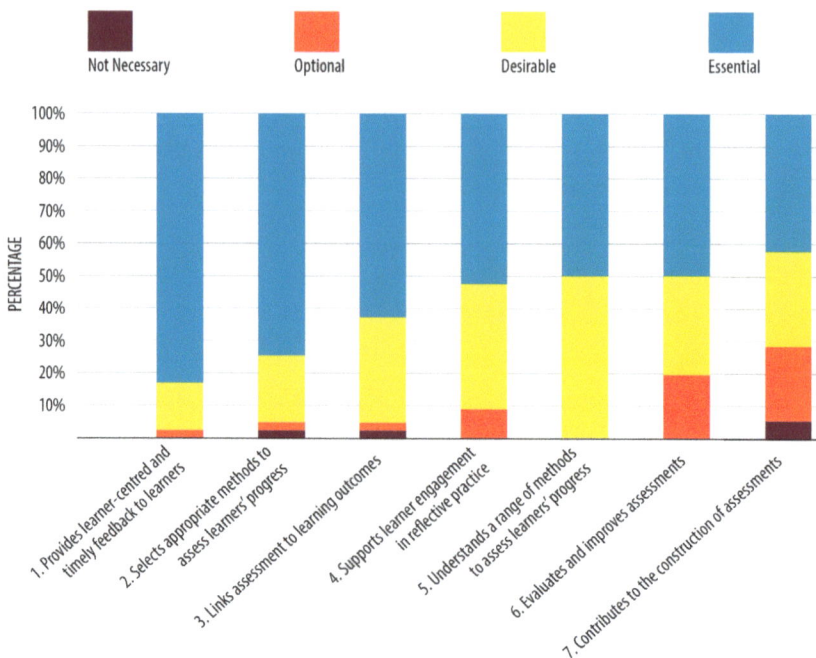

Figure 28: Delphi group Round 1 rating of activities 3 – Learner progression (full axis labels are given in Table 25).

Table 25: Round 1 activities results for learner progression, ordered by mean.

Activities	Desirable/ Essential	Mean	SD	Count
Provides learner-centred and timely feedback to learners	97.2%	3.81	0.46	36
Selects appropriate methods to assess learners' progress	94.4%	3.67	0.67	36
Links assessment to learning outcomes	94.5%	3.56	0.68	36
Understands a range of methods to assess learners' progress	100.0%	3.50	0.50	36
Supports learner engagement in reflective practice	91.7%	3.44	0.64	36
Evaluates and improves assessments	80.6%	3.31	0.78	36
Contributes to the construction of assessments	72.2%	3.08	0.92	36

and research to be near to perfection' and cannot only be the responsibility of educators alone. One person found that more coherence was needed between curriculum developers and people working on assessment methods: 'Often

Table 26: Round 1 comments on learner progression.

Comment	Number of times mentioned
Assessment can be developed by others	3
Feedback is important	1
More coherence needed	1
'Uses', 'can describe or enumerate' instead of understands	1

curriculum dev and assessment methods are done by disconnected groups; key for them to be linked/aligned'. One respondent wanted to stress the importance of providing feedback. Another commented that they would prefer the terms 'uses, can describe, enumerate' instead of 'understands a range of methods to assess learners' progress'. A summary of comments is presented in Table 26.

Activities – Working in teams

In this group, the list comprised:

1. Actively seeks and develops opportunities to enhance interprofessional education.
2. Collaborates with others to support learning and teaching.
3. Positively influences educational culture.
4. Contributes to educational strategy.
5. Uses a wide range of communication strategies to enhance teamwork.
6. Provides timely and effective feedback to colleagues.

Only one activity in this group met the consensus criteria threshold: 'Collaborates with others to support learning and teaching' (mean >3.4). All others had mean values less than 3.4. Responses to these activities were more widely spread. In general, the rating assigned by participants was lower than for the activities in the other lists: if in the previous lists the majority of answers were in the category 'essential', in this list the larger number of participants rated them 'desirable'. In particular, 'Contributes to educational strategy' did not reach the 80% of responses in 'desirable or essential combined' and did not reach the mean threshold (see Figure 29 and Table 27).

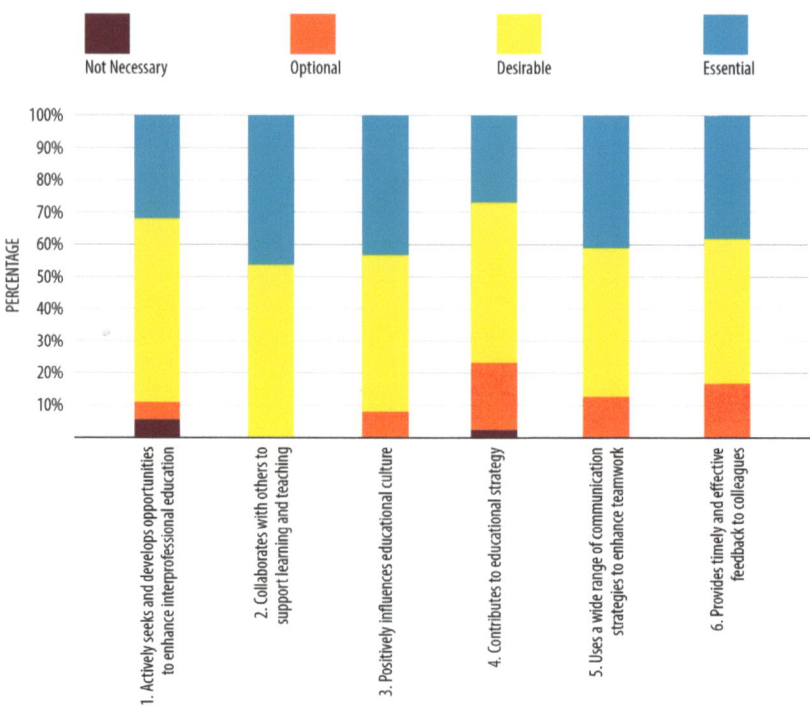

Figure 29: Delphi group Round 1 rating of Activities 4 – Working in teams (full axis labels are given in Table 27).

Table 27: Round 1 activities results for working in teams, ordered by mean.

Activity	Desirable/ Essential	Mean	SD	Count
Collaborates with others to support learning and teaching	100.0%	3.46	0.50	37
Positively influences educational culture	91.9%	3.35	0.62	37
Uses a wide range of communication strategies to enhance teamwork	86.5%	3.27	0.68	37
Provides timely and effective feedback to colleagues	83.8%	3.22	0.70	37
Actively seeks and develops opportunities to enhance interprofessional education	89.2%	3.16	0.75	37
Contributes to educational strategy	75.7%	3.00	0.77	37

Table 28: Round 1 comments on working in teams.

Comment	Number of times mentioned
Teamwork is important	2
Team working is important but with some caveat	3

Comments about working in teams

Five respondents added a comment. Generally, even though the results of the rating are lower than in the other groups of activities, comments concerning activities related to working in teams were positive. Three comments stressed how team working and interprofessional education are important, but with some caveat that it is not 'a panacea for everything' or 'must be done effectively…' because 'not all collaborative educators work well together…'. Table 28 presents a summary of the comments.

Activities – Enhancing quality

In this group, the list comprised:

1. Seeks feedback.
2. Appropriately receives feedback.
3. Reflects and acts on feedback.
4. Undertakes personal professional development to improve educational practice.
5. Evaluates and improves educational activity.
6. Applies research evidence to educational practice.
7. Seeks to share with others the outcomes of their evaluations or innovations.
8. Actively seeks opportunities to use innovative educational approaches.

Two out of the eight activities did not reach the consensus criteria. 'Seeks to share with others the outcomes of their evaluations or innovations' and 'Actively seeks opportunities to use innovative educational approaches' both had means below 3.4 and combined frequency of 'desirable' and 'essential' lower than 80% (see Figure 30 and Table 29).

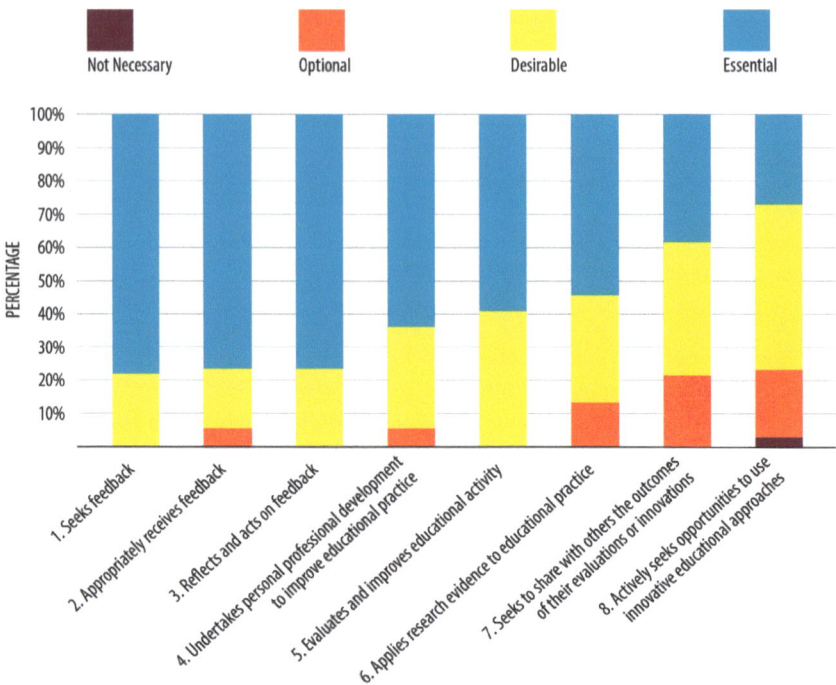

Figure 30: Delphi group Round 1 rating of activities 5 – Enhancing quality (full axis labels are given in Table 29).

Table 29: Round 1 activities results for enhancing quality, ordered by mean.

Activities	Desirable/ Essential	Mean	SD	Count
Seeks feedback	100.0%	3.78	0.41	37
Reflects and acts on feedback	100.0%	3.76	0.43	37
Appropriately receives feedback	94.6%	3.70	0.56	37
Evaluates and improves educational activity	100.0%	3.59	0.49	37
Undertakes personal professional development to improve educational practice	94.6%	3.59	0.59	37
Applies research evidence to educational practice	86.5%	3.41	0.72	37
Seeks to share with others the outcomes of their evaluations or innovations	78.4%	3.16	0.75	37
Actively seeks opportunities to use innovative educational approaches	75.7%	3.00	0.77	37

Table 30: Round 1 comments on enhancing quality.

Comment	Number of times mentioned
Important	3
More important to improve giving feedback	1
Nothing wrong in using tried and trusted methods if they work.	1
More clarity needed on seeking feedback	1
Development is there but not recognised	1

Comments about enhancing quality

Seven respondents added a comment. The majority of comments express the importance of enhancing quality of teaching. Two comments add some concern about feedback: one stresses the need for more clarity in seeking feedback; the other the importance of learning how to give feedback, as 'it is not always constructive…'. Another comment was sceptical about the use of innovative methods as 'nothing wrong in using tried and trusted methods if they work'. About personal development, one comment stressed how most of the time, development is there but not recognised: 'I agree that educators need to undertake development; however, if you get a brand new module and you have to read your way into a whole new subject, these activities are development, without it ever being recognised as such'. A summary of comments is given in Table 30.

Final comments

Five participants left final comments. In general, they were positive about the research. Some expressed a little perplexity about the lists which 'miss the 'edginess' of being an educator'. For example, one commented: 'In some cases the definitions are a bit 'motherhood and apple pie' as in who is going to say that's not a good thing'. Table 31 provides a summary of these comments.

Conclusions from Round 1

Overall there was greater consensus on values compared to activities. Among activities, the items grouped under 'Working in teams' had relatively lower ratings.

Tables 32 and 33 list the items which did not pass the Delphi threshold and were included in Round 2.

Table 31: Round 1 results: Activities – Final comments.

Comment	Number of times mentioned
Good work	4
Good but 'not edgy'	2
Engage learners in meaningful dialogue	1
Recognise changes in learning needs	1
Effective educator is part of the learning process thus has weaknesses and vulnerability	1

Table 32: Value included in second round.

Value	Committed/ Highly Committed	Mean	SD	Count
Interprofessional education	86.5%	3.27	0.76	37

Table 33: Activities included in second round.

Activities – Teaching and supporting learning	Desirable/ Essential	Mean	SD	Count
Uses a range of educational methods and technologies to help students achieve intended learning outcomes	91.9%	3.35	0.62	37
Manages educational resources in a cost-effective manner	89.2%	3.22	0.62	37

Activities – Learner progression	Desirable/ Essential	Mean	SD	Count
Evaluates and improves assessments	80.6%	3.31	0.78	36
Contributes to the construction of assessments	72.2%	3.08	0.92	36

Activities – Working in teams	Desirable/ Essential	Mean	SD	Count
Positively influences educational culture	91.9%	3.35	0.62	37
Uses a wide range of communication strategies to enhance teamwork	86.5%	3.27	0.68	37
Provides timely and effective feedback to colleagues	83.8%	3.22	0.70	37
Actively seeks and develops opportunities to enhance interprofessional education	89.2%	3.16	0.75	37
Contributes to educational strategy	75.7%	3.00	0.77	37

Table 33: *(Contd.)*

Activities – enhancing quality	Desirable/ Essential	Mean	SD	Count
Seeks to share with others the outcomes of their evaluations or innovations	78.4%	3.16	0.75	37
Actively seeks opportunities to use innovative educational approaches	75.7%	3.00	0.77	37

Generally, the comments in all sections contain positive feedback. The most critical positions concern activities that were not considered as main responsibility of the educator (for example, defining learning outcomes, cost management and safety of learners in Table 22 as well as assessment that can be developed by others without lowering the quality of teaching in Table 26).

It is interesting to notice that even if the list of activities in 'Working in teams' were the ones with lower agreement levels, several comments stress that team working is important (see Table 28). The final general 'negative' comment that the lists presented are good but 'not edgy' (Table 31) suggests that they may work well as a baseline threshold for educators.

Round 2 Results

In the second round, participants were asked for feedback on the 12 items which did NOT achieve consensus. For each, they were given the results from Round 1 and invited to submit a second rating.

All Round 1 participants agreed to be contacted again; 33 responded and took part in the second round of the survey.

Values: Round 2 results

In the second round of rating, 'interprofessional education' reached consensus according to the consensus criteria (see Table 34). None of the participants assigned a rating lower than desirable (see Figure 31).

Compared to Round 1, the number of respondents rating committed/highly committed increased from 86.5% to 93.8%. The mean increased from 3.27 to 3.53.

Activities: Round 2 results

According to the consensus criteria, three out of the 11 activities achieved consensus at Round 2 (see Table 35). These are: 'evaluates and improves assessments', 'contributes to the construction of assessments' and 'positively influences educational culture'.

Compared to Round 1 (results also shown in Table 35), although participants assigned higher ratings to all the activities, the means for the remaining eight activities did not meet the consensus criterion. 'Uses a range of educational methods and technologies to help students achieve intended learning outcome' just missed achieving the mean consensus criterion (i.e., mean=3.39). Activity 11, 'Actively seeks opportunities to use innovative educational approaches', was the only item that failed to pass two consensus criteria (the mean <3.4; and for the percentage of combined responses rated as essential/desirable <80%).

Table 34: Round 2 results for value 'Interprofessional education'.

Value (Round 2)	Combined Committed / Highly committed	Mean	SD	Count
Interprofessional education	93.8%	3.53	0.61	32

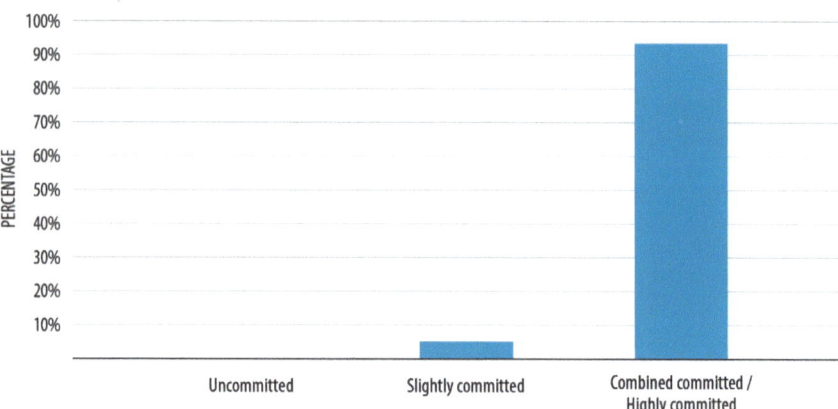

Figure 31: Delphi group Round 2 rating of values.

Table 35: Activities results Round 2 (Round 1 results).

	Activities	Desirable/ Essential	Mean	SD	Count
1	Evaluates and improves assessments	84.4% (80.6%)	3.47 (3.31)	0.75 (0.78)	32 (36)
2	Contributes to the construction of assessments	90.6% (72.2%)	3.44 (3.08)	0.75 (0.92)	32 (36)
3	Positively influences educational culture	90.6% (91.9%)	3.41 (3.35)	0.65 (0.62)	32 (37)
4	Uses a range of educational methods and technologies to help students achieve intended learning outcomes	97.0% (91.9%)	3.39 (3.35)	0.55 (0.62)	33 (37)
5	Uses a wide range of communication strategies to enhance teamwork	90.6% (86.5%)	3.38 (3.27)	0.65 (0.68)	32 (37)

Table 35: *(Contd.)*

6	Provides timely and effective feedback to colleagues	90.6% (83.8%)	3.31 (3.22)	0.63 (0.70)	32 (37)
7	Seeks to share with others the outcomes of their evaluations or innovations	87.5% (78.4%)	3.22 (3.16)	0.65 (0.75)	32 (37)
8	Manages educational resources in a cost-effective manner	93.9% (89.2%)	3.18 (3.22)	0.52 (0.62)	33 (37)
9	Actively seeks and develops opportunities to enhance interprofessional education	87.5% (89.2%)	3.13 (3.16)	0.60 (0.75)	32 (37)
10	Contributes to educational strategy	87.5% (75.7%)	3.09 (3.00)	0.58 (0.77)	32 (37)
11	Actively seeks opportunities to use innovative educational approaches	78.1% (75.7%)	2.94 (3.00)	0.61 (0.77)	32 (37)

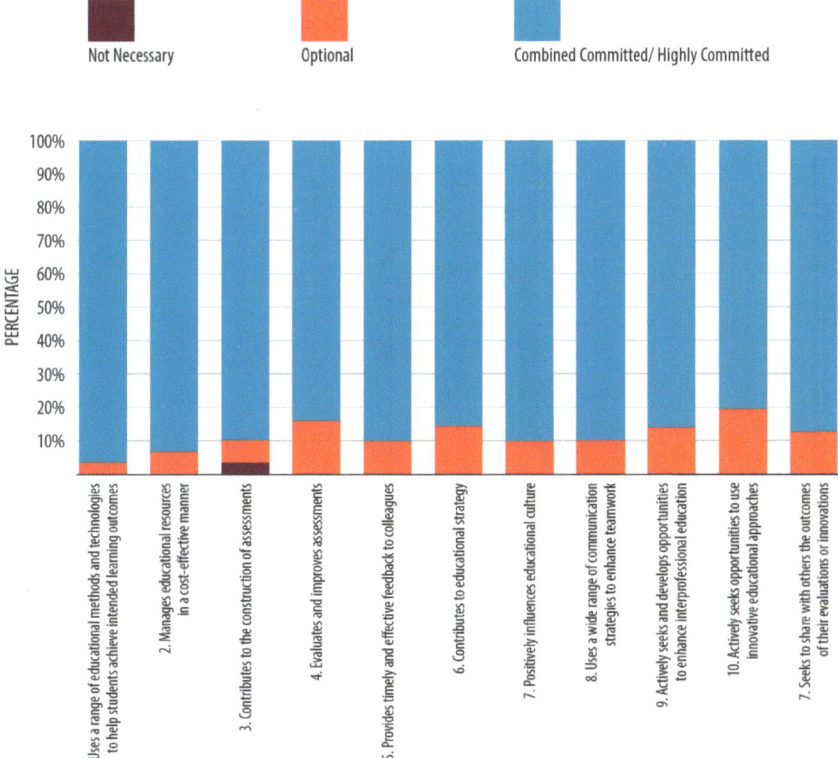

Figure 32: Delphi group Round 2 rating of activities.

Figure 32 shows the distribution of responses for the second round. It is visible how the majority of respondents rated these as desirable/essential (i.e., green bars) although only activities 1 to 3 met the consensus criteria (see Table 35).

Activity 2, 'Contributes to the construction of assessment', was the only item rated not necessary by any participant.

The Final Consensus

The items achieving consensus after two rounds are shown in Tables 36 and 37:

Table 36: Values achieving consensus after two rounds.

Value	Combined Committed / Highly committed	Mean
Ethical conduct	100.0%	3.97
Upholding patient wellbeing and safety	100.0%	3.89
Respect for learners	100.0%	3.78
(High) Quality in education	97.3%	3.76
Fairness	94.6%	3.59
Respect for colleagues	100.0%	3.59
Accountability	94.6%	3.51
Personal development as an educator	94.6%	3.43
Interprofessional education (R2)	93.8%	3.53

Table 37: Activities achieving consensus after two rounds.

Activities *preparation for teaching and learning*	Desirable/ Essential	Mean
Aligns planned activities with the intended learning outcomes	100.0%	3.78
Identifies the learning needs of students	100.0%	3.76
Understands the (changing) context of learning environment (e.g., regulation, workforce)	100.0%	3.65
Understands how principles of teaching and learning are applied to the preparation of teaching	94.6%	3.64
Defines learning outcomes and subject content	97.3%	3.62
Demonstrates an awareness of a range of learning and teaching methods	94.6%	3.57
Makes effective use of resources (human, financial resources and learning technologies)	94.6%	3.43

Table 37: *(contd.)*

Activities *teaching and supporting learning*	**Desirable/ Essential**	**Mean**
Balances the needs of learners with the need to provide safe patient care	100.0%	3.86
Establishes a safe and effective learning environment	100.0%	3.81
Applies principles of adult learning to their teaching practices	91.9%	3.49
Activities *learner progression*	**Desirable/ Essential**	**Mean**
Provides learner-centred and timely feedback to learners	97.2%	3.81
Selects appropriate methods to assess learners' progress	94.4%	3.67
Links assessment to learning outcomes	94.5%	3.56
Understands a range of methods to assess learners' progress	100.0%	3.50
Supports learner engagement in reflective practice	91.7%	3.44
Evaluates and improves assessments (R2)	84.4%	3.47
Contributes to the construction of assessments (R2)	90.6%	3.44
Activities *working in teams*	**Desirable/ Essential**	**Mean**
Collaborates with others to support learning and teaching	100.0%	3.46
Positively influences educational culture (R2)	90.6%	3.41
Activities *enhancing quality*	**Desirable/ Essential**	**Mean**
Seeks feedback	100.0%	3.78
Reflects and acts on feedback	100.0%	3.76
Appropriately receives feedback	94.6%	3.70
Evaluates and improves educational activity	100.0%	3.59
Undertakes personal professional development to improve educational practice	94.6%	3.59
Applies research evidence to educational practice	86.5%	3.41

Endnotes

(1) 1=uncommitted, 2=slightly committed, 3=committed, 4=highly committed.
(2) Thirty-seven respondents rated the first section (values), but some of the activity items were rated by 36 only.

CHAPTER 7

Conclusions

Limitations

In this concluding section we describe some key discussions that arose during the development of the descriptors of values and activities (DVAs) and explain in more detail how these were resolved. Our discussion of these issues should be understood in the context of a number of limitations to our study. We were challenged to find source documents – standards and guidance for all healthcare professions – and although we tracked down over 50 in the end, not all were relevant and some may have been missed, especially where these did not have English translations. Inevitably the greatest number of standards documents came from medicine and nursing; this is hardly surprising given the size of each profession and the diversity of specialties within those professions: however, our subsequent analysis was not based on frequency but on themes, which meant that the number of documents or their professional origin had little bearing on the final analysis. While we endeavoured to ensure maximum representation from all healthcare professions (HCPs), unsurprisingly the largest professions (doctors and nurses) were among the most numerous and vocal respondents. In addition, the nature of the study meant that only those with a strong interest in the subject (either negative or favourable) were likely to participate, which may have affected the results. We struggled to engage the smaller professions and where only one or two individual healthcare educators' (HCE) views were gathered from small healthcare specialties, there was an increased risk that their views were given undue weight.

This was mitigated to a large extent by the multi-methods approach. In addition, the research team are non-clinical healthcare educators, which reduced the risk of possible bias in favour of a particular HCP; data collection and analysis were invariably carried out by two or more members of the

---

How to cite this book chapter:
Browne, J., Bullock, A., Parker, S., Poletti, C., Jenkins, J., and Gallen, D. 2021. Conclusions. *Educators of Healthcare Professionals: Agreeing a Shared Purpose*. Pp. 95–104. Cardiff, UK: Cardiff University Press. DOI: https://doi.org/10.18573/book6.g. License: CC-BY-NC-ND

team and independently checked by other team members; and results were carefully triangulated.

We were aware when we started the work that there was a degree of scepticism in some areas about the feasibility of the task we had been set. In particular, there was some concern that achieving a consensus on values and activities that would be acceptable to a wide group of professions at varying levels of proficiency would result in a set of descriptors so bland and minimal that they were of limited use. We are pleased to note that this has not proved to be the case, thanks to the educational expertise, insight and engagement of our respondents. We report some of the key discussions here and show how some apparently contradictory viewpoints were resolved within the study.

Conceptualising Generic DVAs

During all stages of the research, there were a number of ongoing debates about what may reasonably be expected of every educator, and how these expectations may be expressed in unambiguous terms when in practice there is considerable variation. There were five key 'fault lines' where the overall weight of opinion needed to be balanced carefully to ensure that the final DVAs selected were genuinely reflective of the best aspects of all HCEs' work while not making them too ambitious or idealistic to be relevant.

1. Descriptive versus aspirational

Some respondents saw the DVAs as an opportunity to drive up educational quality by setting them at a level that might require some HCEs to undertake additional professional development. For example, some respondents felt that high-quality clinical supervision required background understanding of educational theory. Others, however, argued that it was possible for an individual clinical supervisor to instinctively be a good mentor without being able to describe clearly the theoretical principles of workplace-based assessment and feedback, and that requiring a knowledge of educational theory would exclude and alienate many excellent practitioners.

This reflects a wider debate within healthcare education. Nearly all HCPs are expected to supervise, assess and mentor students and trainees. At the same time, it is widely acknowledged that healthcare education theory, research and practice also constitute a specialty in its own right, leading some HCEs to undertake advanced postgraduate studies and develop significant academic and management careers in the field. Even where HCEs do not expect to make education a significant part of their career, many voluntarily undertake additional CPD as part of their commitment to clinical excellence. The point at which an HCE should be expected to *start* acquiring specialist educational knowledge and skills, however, is not clear and varies between professions.

Some professions mandate educational theory and practice as part of basic undergraduate training with clear skills development throughout an individual's career; but others, as we have observed, require no training at all, or expect HCEs to undertake basic training only on being appointed to educational roles (Austerberry & Newman 2013). It may therefore be reasonable for one profession to expect that all HCEs within that profession should understand some basic principles of educational design, where another might view this as a more specialist responsibility.

In attempting to resolve this debate, we felt it important to emphasise that the aim of this project was to produce generic DVAs. Where such issues arose in open discussion, therefore, the researchers reminded participants of this aim. Ultimately most respondents took the pragmatic view that the final outputs needed to be relevant, applicable and useful to all healthcare educators (HCE) without exception and regardless of level of seniority or profession. The outcome of this therefore is that the DVAs are descriptive rather than developmental; it would be up to individual professions to stipulate any additional profession-specific requirements.

> KEY PRINCIPLE 1: All HCEs, regardless of level of seniority or profession, will be able to engage with all DVAs.

2. Knows versus does

In some cases, items were treated ambiguously depending on how participants in our study conceived the expected level of engagement on the part of the HCE. In the domain of teaching and supporting learning, for example, some participants in both the nominal group and the workshop felt that HCEs, especially those at an early level of their careers, might well be using other people's educational material rather than material they have developed themselves. These respondents argued that early career educators did not therefore need to know how to *develop* teaching and learning resources. Others felt that regardless of this, all HCEs would normally be expected to know how the material they are using was developed in order to be able to critique and improve it, and the DVAs should reflect this expectation.

Similar issues were raised in phases 4 and 5 regarding learner progression, where it was argued that many HCEs' involvement is limited to the administration of tests designed by others. Again, the consensus view appeared to be that regardless of whether individual educators selected or designed the assessment themselves, they still would be expected to be able to explain the educational rationale, technical design and key features to learners.

This would reflect the general principle applied to the development of the DVAs, that even where an individual was either: (a) not currently engaged in a particular activity, or (b) not personally responsible for the selection, design, development or evaluation of that activity, they should be able to explain it to learners and other stakeholders and use their knowledge of it as a way of informing their educational practice.

> KEY PRINCIPLE 2: All activities require understanding to the extent that the practitioner can explain the purpose, process and outcome of that activity to key stakeholders (e.g., learners, colleagues and patients).

3. Value versus activity

Some further questions were raised where an item was viewed as ambiguous because it was not clear if it was a value or an activity.

For example, some respondents felt that interprofessional education (IPE) is an activity. At the same time, it was acknowledged that not only are some HCEs not involved in IPE but others, possibly due to local factors, never have the opportunity to undertake it. This was an argument for excluding it. But others felt that it is a value, and thus it is reasonable to expect that all HCEs should be committed to it regardless of their ability to participate in it.

Similarly, an early item – fairness in admissions, involving a commitment to widening participation and diversity – was also viewed ambiguously. The admissions part was eventually dropped while the commitment to fairness was retained.

Thus, as we worked through these practical issues, a further general principle was applied to the development of the DVAs. Where an item achieved consensus, but it was not clear if it was a value or an activity, that item would be viewed as a value requiring commitment but not necessarily practical participation.

> KEY PRINCIPLE 3: All values require commitment to the extent that the practitioner can explain how their values inform their educational practice.

4. Leadership – individual versus collective

There was a complex debate about whether certain educational activities should apply to all HCEs regardless of seniority. Was it reasonable to expect every HCE to engage with some items such as leadership and quality, or should these apply only to a subset of specialist educators who had developed advanced expertise in a particular activity or who occupied more senior roles?

Leadership was especially problematic because, as with IPE, there was disagreement about whether it is a value or an activity. Those treating it as a value argued that one may be committed to and support good leadership and management while not necessarily being in a senior role oneself. As a value, it would apply to all HCEs. Others argued that leadership and management were activities, leading to further significant debate about whether all HCEs should be involved in or aspire to leadership. Some groups of respondents viewed leadership as a generic skill that all HCEs, regardless of seniority, should be able to demonstrate – this idea of leadership as a universal responsibility aligns with the concept of 'collective leadership' (West et al. 2015). Others felt strongly that to assert this diminished the status of leadership as a unique set of practices and understandings that could be acquired through experiential learning and further study. They argued that leadership was a specialist high-level skill that required additional development only for a sub-group of HCEs. The greater the level of seniority of the respondents, the more divisive this question appeared to be.

Discussion of dimensions of leadership (such as change management, resource use, quality improvement and quality assurance) also reflected this divide in thinking between (a) those who felt that these items were the responsibility of those in leadership roles; and (b) those who felt there needed to be a more collective understanding of the role all educators play in advancing clinical education and improving clinical care through their proactive work in developing tomorrow's HCPs.

The development and presentation of the DVAs have been informed by this debate in the following ways:

(a) Leadership and management are not a separate domain, reflecting the view that not all HCPs occupy or aspire to educational leadership roles.
(b) The DVAs reflect a broader contemporary understanding of collective leadership within the wider healthcare education team. Elements associated with leadership such as collaborative working, use of resources and interprofessional education are therefore retained. These are areas where HCEs often find themselves called upon to demonstrate leadership regardless of seniority, particularly when working with non-educator colleagues, patients, students and the public.

> KEY PRINCIPLE 4: All HCEs, regardless of level of seniority or profession, participate in collective leadership within the wider healthcare education team.

5. Employer versus individual

During the literature review, a number of 'standards' and 'guidance' documents, ostensibly for HCEs, were excluded when it became apparent that their focus was at the institutional level (e.g., WFME 2015). Such documents often set minimum standards for teaching rooms, documentation, induction and training processes and so on, which were not in themselves under the control of individual HCEs. Our brief was to focus on the individual HCE rather than the employing institution, but when exploring the literature, it was occasionally hard to make this distinction; when such issues occurred, the research team conferred and reached a collective decision.

This conceptual divide persisted and became evident on a number of occasions, particularly during the INHWE workshop feedback, where issues such as 'fairness in admissions', 'use of resources' and 'stakeholder engagement' were seen by some to be matters for institutions to address rather than the individual responsibility of the HCEs. One group at the INHWE meeting identified 17 such items, placing them in a category which they named 'Programme Governance' – again, further recognition that for some educators, their daily practice is heavily proscribed by the environment and institutions in which they teach.

Nevertheless, the point of identifying HCE DVAs is to acknowledge the significant role played by individual educators in the support and delivery of safe and effective healthcare education. While they cannot do this without the support of the institutions and organisations for which they work, they, like all clinical staff, have a duty of candour – a responsibility to ensure their work is of a high standard and to take action to address conditions where they cannot perform in a safe and effective manner. This is particularly important where teaching is taking place with patients present. It is essential that all HCEs are committed to balancing effective education with the need to ensure patient safety and high-quality patient care. HCEs are professionals and this means that this responsibility may not be 'outsourced' to the institutions for which they work.

As a result of this understanding, the DVAs acknowledge within their structure the ethical responsibility of all HCEs to actively ensure safe and effective learning and teaching for the benefit, not just of the individual learners, but also of their patients.

KEY PRINCIPLE 5: All HCEs actively ensure safe and effective learning and teaching for the benefit of patients as well as learners.

Organisational Structure

Our intention from the outset was to leave organising the DVAs into domains until as late as possible in the research process, since the individual items needed to be discussed independently of each other. We accepted that it would eventually be necessary to organise a set of up to 40 DVAs into domains to make them more manageable and useful; but we were reasonably confident that these domains would emerge naturally during the research process, and this proved to be the case.

The nominal group was particularly helpful in this regard, collapsing several activities into 'efficient and effective learning and teaching', and a number of values-based items into 'professionalism' and 'communication'. The way in which domain groupings were suggested, modified and discarded was useful in demonstrating the benefits of labelling each domain in a manner that showed a clear connection between the items.

The INHWE meeting was also helpful; the DVAs were presented in alphabetical order with no distinction made between values and activities. As a result of this exercise, a number of issues were highlighted including: the conflicting ideas around what items were seen in terms of both value and activity; the challenges around what level of engagement could reasonably be expected from all HCEs; and the lack of distinction between what could reasonably be expected of an individual and what was the responsibility of the organisation.

Final Domain Groupings

The Delphi group were presented with loose groupings of DVAs, and it was here that the final central values plus four domains were determined: VALUES at the centre, with PREPARATION FOR TEACHING AND LEARNING, TEACHING AND SUPPORTING LEARNING, LEARNER PROGRESSION and QUALITY ranged around them in a roughly temporal order (see Figure 33).

The justification for organising the DVAs both thematically and temporally is that they reflect the actual teaching process and its cyclical nature.

Central values

Good educators begin and end with their professional values, and everything they do is in support of and informed by these.

(1) Preparation for teaching

Good educators prepare for their teaching in advance wherever possible, ensuring that they understand and can explain clearly the nature, purpose and expected outcomes of every contact session with learners.

(2) Teaching and supporting learning

During teaching sessions, good educators pay attention to the learning environment, ensuring it is safe and productive for all involved, including learners, patients and colleagues. They make it their responsibility to offer learners the best possible learning opportunities, working in teams where necessary to ensure high quality teaching and learning.

(3) Learner progression

Good educators monitor and assess learners' progress both during and after teaching sessions, ensuring that feedback is prompt, accurate and useful to learners. They help learners to understand and reflect on the feedback they have received, and to take appropriate remedial action where necessary.

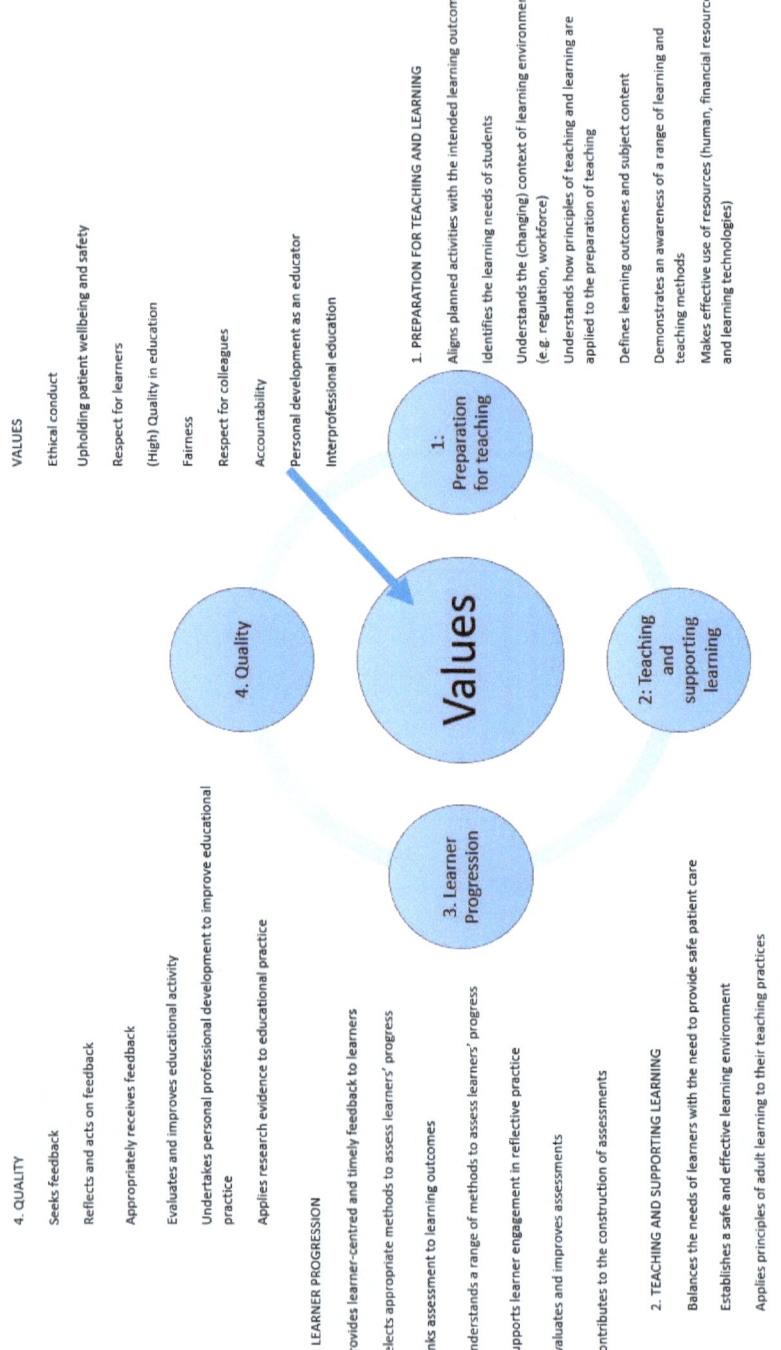

Figure 33: The descriptors of the 9 value and 24 activities, organised by domain.

(4) Quality

Good educators are mindful of their own practice as educators, evaluating their own practice, seeking feedback, using evidence to improve their performance and keeping their own skills up to date. They reflect on their practice as educators and use their reflections to make continuous improvements both to their individual practice and, where possible, in the wider educational setting.

Taken in turn, active participation in each domain, if it is informed and driven by professional values, should lead the user naturally through a continuous improvement cycle (Figure 34). Change will inevitably take place as the educator works through a cycle of 'prepare to teach (plan), reflection-in-action during teaching (do), reflection-on-action after teaching (study), design improvement (act)'.

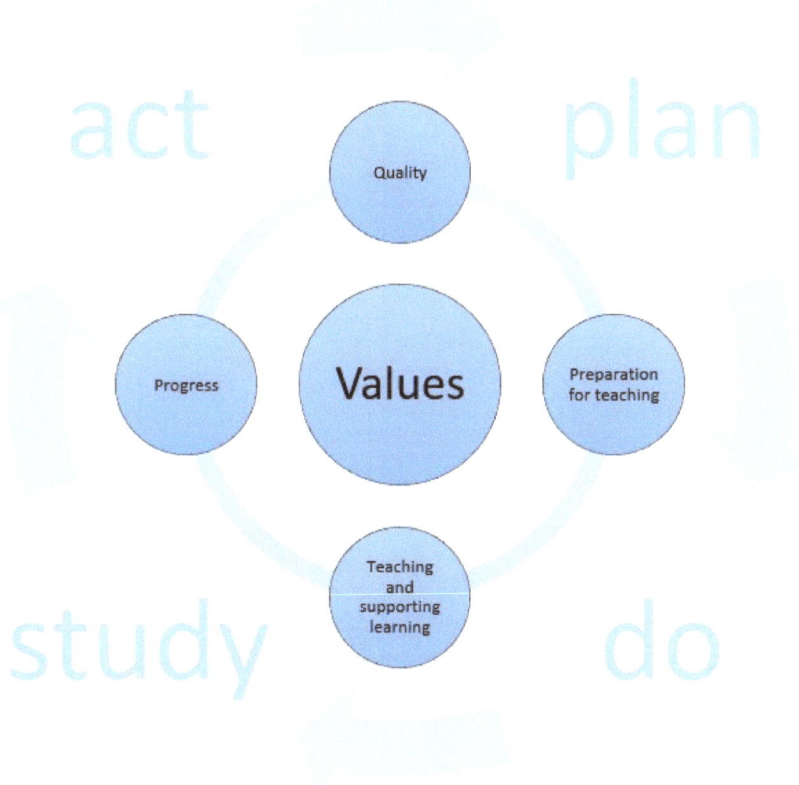

Figure 34: How the DVA framework supports continuous quality improvement.

The benefit to those using the DVA framework is that over time, the individual will be expected to make progress, building on their basic skills to develop their profile within their own specialty. Figure 35 is a lively and light-hearted sketch, expertly drawn by Laura Sorvala, showing the dynamic interaction of the HEVA framework to support individuals in a beneficial learning cycle. The optimistic upward spiral represents the positive progress educators can make if they regularly plan, do, review and improve their teaching and learning practices against the HEVA framework.

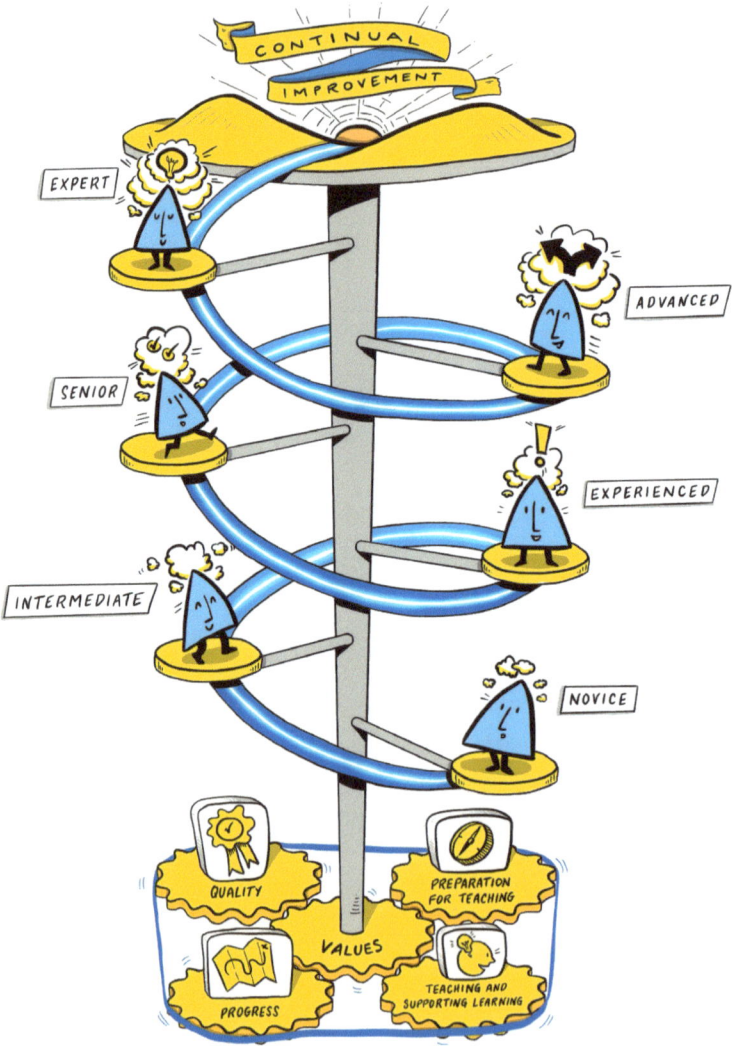

Figure 35: How the DVA Framework supports educator progression (image, Laura Sorvala).

CHAPTER 8

The Way Forward

The effective delivery of safe and high-quality healthcare increasingly requires complex, context-dependent distributed cognition, skills and behaviours, to support the team-based delivery of care (Holt et al. 2010; Thistlethwaite et al. 2014; Uhling et al. 2018). Such interprofessional ways of working are being increasingly recognised as essential in the UK, if health services are to better respond to the challenges facing them (AoMRC et al. 2017). This has been highlighted in a range of recent documents, including the *Five Year Forward View – Next Steps* (NHS England) and the *NHS Long Term Plan* (NHS UK 2019). It has also been noted by a range of individual healthcare profession regulators and by the UK Professional Standards Authority in its role of regulatory oversight. This reflects developments which are significantly more advanced in North America and, though to a lesser extent, in Europe. In Canada, Accreditation of Interprofessional Health Education (AIPHE) argue that: 'IPE is one of the vital strategies that education programs can employ to prepare health care providers to participate in a new, more collaborative, future health care workforce'(AIPHE 2014: 19).

All of this provides the background to the need for a fresh initiative, involving all of the healthcare professions, for a much greater focus on how we can (and should) be educating, training and preparing individuals and teams to develop and implement working practices which are built around shared values and activities instead of our professional silos and jealousies. Such tribalism has been identified as a significant factor in the failure of professional education by Frenk et al. (2010), who argue for a redesign of health professions education. While this has been discussed widely and internationally, there is limited evidence that it is resulting in significant change in attitudes or practice within those responsible for all aspects of healthcare education and training across the United Kingdom and Ireland.

How to cite this book chapter:
Browne, J., Bullock, A., Parker, S., Poletti, C., Jenkins, J., and Gallen, D. 2021. The Way Forward. *Educators of Healthcare Professionals: Agreeing a Shared Purpose.* Pp. 105–116. Cardiff, UK: Cardiff University Press. DOI: https://doi.org/10.18573/book6.h. License: CC-BY-NC-ND

Our study adds constructively to the academic foundation by establishing a consensus across a wide range of healthcare professions regarding a common set of values and activities. There was considerable scepticism at the outset that this work would be impossible owing to the many disparities between healthcare professions, the historical tendency of healthcare professions organisations to communicate primarily within their own traditional groupings, and the evidence that each profession tends to educate its own educators to teach only its own students and trainees. This work has shown that it is, in fact, possible to reach consensus on a set of generic values and activities which can be applied to healthcare educators at all levels across a wide range of professions. As a result of this, it can now be argued more authoritatively that, at least for educators in the healthcare professions, we have far more in common than was previously thought. Moreover, many traditional dividing lines have been shown to be due more to terminology and linguistic usages than any real-world differences.

The primary implications of this are threefold. First, it is important that these DVAs are brought to the attention of those with responsibilities in this area and used to develop unified expectations of all those performing roles as educators of healthcare professionals. Secondly, further study is needed to explore how these DVAs may be used in practice; we hypothesise that there may be considerable strategic benefits to aligning the professional development of NHS HCEs across the board. Third, there will be knock-on benefits to HCPs as they work to identify and establish those additional activities and areas of knowledge that are unique to their own educators. One further benefit to HPE organisations is that they will be able to identify and mandate the additional specialty-specific skills and knowledge required of their HCEs as they progress towards more senior roles with wider levels of responsibility.

The benefits to individual HCEs are likely to include greater clarity about the expectations of their role, reassurance that their values and activities are common to and recognised by all HCPs, and increased confidence regarding their ability to work across traditional professional boundaries.

The Complexities of Interprofessional Teaching and Learning

CAIPE's definition of interprofessional learning – 'Students learning with, from and about each other' – is so useful, it has become the favoured phrase to describe this type of learning (Barr 2002).

But as a definition of what takes place during the activity of interprofessional education, it has one glaring omission: it completely omits the teacher from the activity. While one may legitimately argue that an educator does not need to be present for interprofessional learning to take place, there perhaps needs to be a further refinement of how interprofessional teaching is regarded that takes account of the fundamental role of the teacher in conceiving, designing, preparing, supporting and assessing the effectiveness of the learning opportunity, whether physically present or not. For while definitions of interprofessional education are quite rightly student-centred, the role of the educator is nevertheless not insignificant: it is a major factor in the success or failure of IPE (Steinert 2005).

Institutions, regulators, managers and employers have always predicated their educational policies on trust – they rely heavily on the expectation that the individual educator is competent to teach. While this assumption has proved to be dangerously false in some cases (Clarke et al. 2012; Monrouxe et al. 2015), the majority of healthcare educators are at least able to teach, supervise and assess learners within their own professional group in the workplace without significant detriment to the junior practitioner or risk to patient care. Indeed, in many cases teaching is effective and even inspiring, producing trained clinicians who have the necessary skills, knowledge and attitudes to practise safely (Gunderman 2006).

Individual professions' confidence in the basic teaching competence of most of their practitioners (albeit with an understanding that teaching skills can always be improved) would appear to be reasonably well justified where teaching involves an educator who is teaching learners within their own profession as in Figure 36. It is important to note that the figure is simplified to represent a transmission model of education with the teacher at the top. We appreciate that this may not represent the reality of healthcare education, which more often relies on a flatter hierarchy, with communication going in both directions.

Regulators, institutions and organisations monitor the progress of their graduates and licentiates and there is no solid evidence that academic and performance standards are falling. Many may also mandate training and supervision for their educators, but they usually concern themselves only with the performance and progress of those working and learning within the single professional groups for which they are responsible. So far, so good; while there is always room for improvement, individual professions have a good grasp on the education and training of their junior members and many also have a clear idea of what a good educator within their profession should look like.

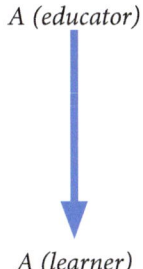

A (educator)

A (learner)

Figure 36: Educator from profession A teaches learner or learners from profession A. Solid line indicates formal communication (knowledge transfer) between paired professional groups.

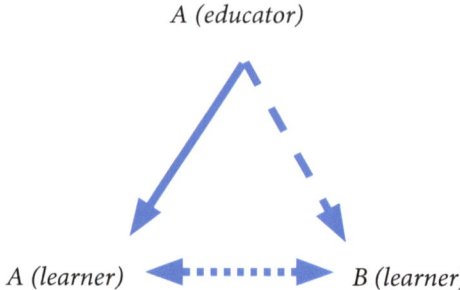

Figure 37: Educator from profession A teaches learner or learners from professions A and B.

Figure 37, however, shows how even a modest attempt to introduce an element of interprofessional education adds an additional level of risk and complexity that is often not acknowledged. As in Figure 36, the solid line indicates formal communication (knowledge transfer) between paired professional groups (A to A). The dashed line indicates formal communication (instruction) between teachers and learners from unpaired professional groups (in this case, profession A to profession B), while the dotted line indicates informal communication (such as discussion, social communication and problem solving) between unpaired professional groups (A to B and B to A).

In the example shown in Figure 37, normally seen as the first step in interprofessional education, the educator is working with learners from their own profession (A) along with learners from profession B. The complexity comes from the requirement for the educator to communicate on an equal footing with both groups while at the same time fostering effective inter-group communication. The educator may feel reasonably comfortable with teaching learners from their own professional group, but will face challenges both in understanding the expectations and needs of the learners in group B and in facilitating learning conversations between the two disparate groups of learners. The educator will need to be particularly careful to avoid any perception on either side that learners in group A have an advantage, because an essential element in IPE is role modelling fairness and respect within the team, regardless of profession. In this model, the educational organiser or regulator for the learners in group B is taking it on trust that an educator from profession A is able to teach them to the same standards and levels of competence that would be expected of an educator from profession B. But this, as we have repeatedly shown throughout this book, may not be the case.

There is a significant accentuation of complexity and risk inherent in Figure 38, where an educator from profession A is teaching learners from professions B and C. In this case the educator does not share a professional identity with any of the learners. As before, the dashed lines indicate formal

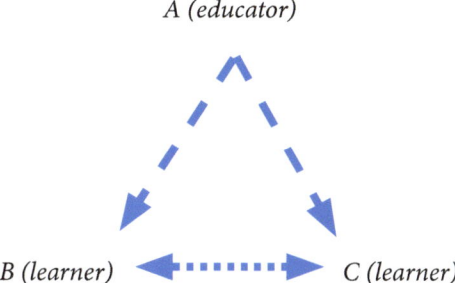

Figure 38: Educator from profession A teaches learner or learners from professions B and C.

communication (instruction) between unpaired professional groups (A to B and A to C) and the dotted line indicates informal communication between unpaired professional groups (B to C and C to B).

In dealing with groups of learners, educators need to remain authentic – communicating honestly and openly, admitting to faults and errors that led to learning – while also retaining credibility as an experienced professional (Molloy & Bearman 2019). This is a difficult tightrope to walk at the best of times. In the scenario shown in Figure 38, this challenge is heightened because the educator cannot rely on the learners' familiarity with (and respect for) his or her professional background, and because the educator is expected to facilitate constructive learning conversations between two other professional groups with whom the educator may have limited experience. Yet this is a fairly typical interprofessional learning scenario in some universities and colleges of healthcare. In this scenario both of the education organisers responsible for the learners in profession B and profession C are assuming that the educator from profession A is competent to teach them. Yet, in reality, they may have no real idea of the extent to which the educator (the product of a teacher training system almost entirely focussed on the education of students from profession A) is qualified to do so.

As we observed in chapter 1, theories of interprofessional education suggest that it will have the maximum effect and will work most effectively where a team of educators comes together to create an active learning experience for interprofessional groups of learners (Burgess et al. 2020). This approach to the organisation and delivery of IPE would therefore produce a scenario closer to that of Figure 4. In this simplified model educators from three different professions are educating learners from three different professions.

The astonishing complexity and multiple challenges of the task facing the interprofessional educators in the scenario depicted in Figure 39 now become clear. Only two of the learners' professions overlap with the educators' professions. Each educator is managing communication with other individuals,

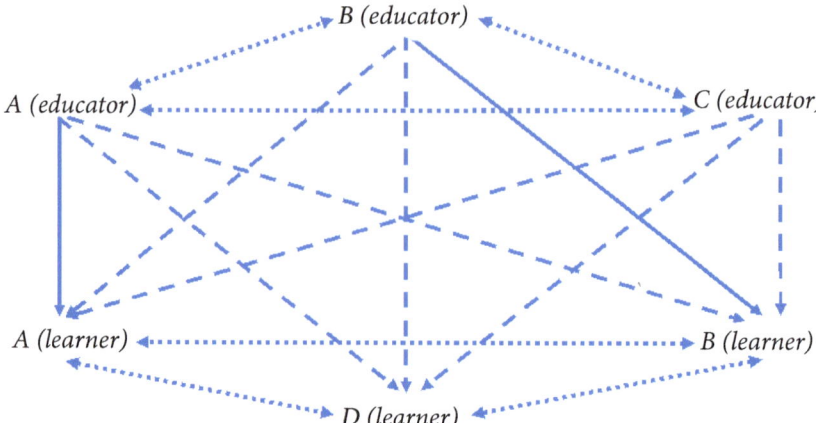

Figure 39: Educators from professions A, B and C teach learners from professions A, B and D.

both teachers and learners, from a different profession. Each group of learners is interacting with at least two educators and two other groups of learners with whom shared understandings and attitudes both about healthcare and about education may not be taken for granted. In Figure 39, there is nobody on the educator team or even within the learner group with whom educator C shares a professional background or identity. The risks involved (of misunderstandings and miscommunication resulting from lack of information, traditional prejudices and the other barriers to IPE that were discussed in more detail in chapter 1) are high for everyone in the group, but particularly so for educator C. And for the learners from profession D, there is nobody with whom they share a professional identity.

The risks inherent in this scenario are obvious. While there may be good will and even educational competence in each professional group and individual, team competence – the glue that sticks learning and teaching teams together so that they can operate effectively – cannot be taken for granted. Yet this is precisely what each profession's educational managers and leaders are assuming when mandating IPE for their learners. Moreover, they are also taking it on trust that other professional groups' teachers are fully equipped to teach their learners, when, as Yvonne Steinert points out (2005):

> most teachers are products of an educational system whose perspective is limited to that of their own discipline. The majority did not train in an interprofessional environment and many do not practice with one another. As a result, teachers may be either uncomfortable with this approach to teaching and learning, or not sufficiently knowledgeable to teach within it.

How a Common Framework Can Lead to Educational Improvements

Educator identity revisited

There is, however, one significant but often overlooked factor that could make a major difference in how the interprofessional teaching team is able to overcome professional barriers. That is, as we have consistently argued throughout this book, the degree to which the educators have a shared understanding of the values and activities that underpin their work. It is this shared understanding that will enable each member of the teaching team to self-identify as a healthcare educator, and that will contribute strongly to their motivation and ability to work with other educators regardless of primary professional background.

We have shown that at present, this shared understanding may not be taken for granted and that each profession has its own perspective on what a good educator within that profession should know, do and value *within that profession's educational practice*. Yet at the same time, our work has shown how much overlap there is between professions. This central area of overlap must be built on to provide the foundation on which educators from all healthcare professions can develop a shared professional identity – that of healthcare educator.

An Early Start to Educator Identity Development

The focus of our work so far has been on identifying and achieving consensus on the baseline values and activities that all educators share. It would be gratifying to think that all educators are working to the basic standards reflected in the HEVA framework, but this is unlikely to be the case in view of the number of reports of educational shortcomings that appear so often in the literature (for example, Fullerton et al. 2019; Knapp et al. 2014; McCrann, Flitcroft & Loughman 2020; Russell & Foulkes 2019). Despite widespread concern about standards in healthcare education, few professions have as yet risen to the challenge of mandating basic educational skills and knowledge as a condition of primary qualification. A coherent core curriculum on education for all undergraduate health professions students would go a long way towards addressing the widespread deficiencies in educational skills among healthcare practitioners which are at the root of these problems – such as inappropriate treatment of students, inadequate teaching in classrooms and clinical settings, poorly defined and assessed learning outcomes and so on. These issues are rarely unique to any single profession but cut right across the healthcare professions education spectrum.

Research has plainly shown that despite the expectation that all clinicians will teach, supervise, appraise and assess colleagues, early career clinicians struggle to assimilate the role of healthcare educator into the professional identity that they acquire during their primary professional training (as, for example, a pharmacist, audiologist or paramedic) (Aguayo Gonzalez & Monereo 2012; Burton, Boschmans & Hoelson 2013; Neese 2003; Sabel et al. 2014). Many clinicians will never acquire this perspective on the importance to patient care of high-quality professional education. Of these, some will nevertheless teach diligently, developing skills and attitudes as they go, but many will continue to view education and educational CPD as an irritating additional responsibility that takes them away from their 'proper job' of patient care and service delivery. These are likely to teach reluctantly or without interest or expertise, and without basic educational skills will remain stuck in the same teaching rut in which they themselves were taught, while unable or unwilling to improve their proficiency (Dahlstrom et al. 2005).

This lack of basic understanding of the fundamental imperative for all clinicians to be willing and able to participate in training future generations of healthcare professions results from the negative hidden curriculum of undergraduate healthcare. A student who has not been prepared to teach effectively at the point of graduation will struggle to accept that teaching is a central part of the role – and therefore the identity – of all healthcare practitioners. It is vital that schools of healthcare and universities begin to respond to this challenge *while students' professional identities are being formed*; at present the lack of teaching and education content within undergraduate healthcare curricula makes engaging early career practitioners in developing educational interests so much harder than it needs to be (Amorosa, Mellman & Graham 2011).

The HEVA framework, because it contains a distillation of what each healthcare profession deems important in education, is perfectly placed to provide a basic interprofessional curriculum through which all students, regardless of primary professional discipline, can share learning.

The Basis for Educational Excellence

Our work also needs to be seen in the light of the need to continue to develop experts and leaders in healthcare education. While it is frequently understood that healthcare education is something that all health professionals should do as a routine part of their job, it is also clear from our work that healthcare education can be – and indeed for some practitioners, is – much more than that.

Much work has gone into exploring the challenges faced by clinicians and academics who aspire to senior roles in healthcare education, and these would appear to be common to all healthcare professions. The most frequently cited barriers include: unclear career paths (Browne, Webb & Bullock 2018), lack of time to teach (Spencer 2003), difficulty with selecting and gaining access to high-quality teacher training (Schoening 2013), shortage of and difficulty identifying role models (Draugalis et al. 2006), high clinical workload (Leggate & Russell 2002), poor or absent recognition and reward schemes (Dybowski &

Harendza 2014) and, most damagingly of all, the perception that teaching is of low priority compared to research or service delivery (Sabel et al. 2014).

Despite education and training of junior clinicians and students having taken place since the time of Hippocrates, healthcare education has yet to achieve the status of a discipline or specialty in its own right (Browne 2021). This is a strange state of affairs in view of the complex skills, advanced knowledge and specialist expertise that senior healthcare educators must develop during their careers. Part of the problem, we would argue, is that healthcare education has been hiding in plain sight for so long.

By this, we mean that most healthcare professionals are able to point to at least one teacher or colleague who is an outstanding educator, who is a role model for students and trainees, who has advanced knowledge of educational theory, who is active in quality improvement and educational audit, and so on, but very few are able to define clearly what an excellent educator knows, does and believes. And while defining excellence in healthcare education remains nebulous, achieving it and measuring it will be impossible (Crosby & Harden 2000). While our work has shown that mono-professional standards are in the process of development in most health professions, recognition of the outstanding work of educators in healthcare across and between all disciplines, levels and types of learner will be slow in coming until there is a much broader consensus that covers the education of all health professions (Browne 2021).

Standards are sometimes viewed as a blunt instrument, enforcing a narrow and rigid approach to professional development that focuses on 'competence' rather than 'excellence'. This does not need to be the case. Assessment drives learning, so it is not the standards themselves which force a focus on competence but the way they are assessed in practice. Assessment methods which meet Van Der Vleuten and Schuwirth's tests for utility (2005) and which emphasise validity through performance in practice would ensure such standards were acceptable and respected.

Standards and frameworks, where they have been developed carefully through consultation and rigorously tested, have much to offer in the move to improve and professionalise healthcare education across the board. For healthcare education to achieve a similar professional standing to other types of specialist practice, certain provisions would need to be in place. These provisions can only do their work of professionalisation effectively if they are built on agreed performance standards to which all healthcare educators can adhere.

For healthcare education to achieve the degree of professionalisation across the health and social care spectrum which would raise its standing, so that it becomes an essential skill for every clinician as well as an important healthcare specialty, the following are needed:

Publicly available standards by which the professional activity and performance of healthcare educators can be evaluated: a clear statement of standards and guidance against which individual educators may be objectively assessed by their peers.

High-level training through which those who want to develop healthcare education as a significant professional role can develop the advanced knowledge and skills they need. The HEVA framework is a statement of basic generic values and activities across all professions but more work is needed to look beyond it to the move advanced generic skills required of more senior healthcare educators.

An evidence base: there are many journals and books offering evidence for 'what works' in healthcare education but nearly all focus on education within one profession. There is also literature on interprofessional education which focuses specifically on that particular specialist area of practice. But there is not yet a corpus of literature within healthcare education which speaks to the needs of all educators regardless of primary discipline – and there is not likely to be until such time as all professions agree on the generic standards that apply to all healthcare educators.

Career paths: each profession has its own mechanisms for developing, recognising and promoting healthcare educators but these vary considerably. For most HCPs, becoming a teacher requires further levels of commitment, experience and study, often undefined; promotion is not inevitable or systematic, and progress usually depends on individuals moving from post to post. Standards offer recruiters and managers a clear way to establish how far an individual has progressed in their educator development and solid evidence of achievement that can be recognised and rewarded.

A common understanding of what is shared; common standards would provide a means for professions to identify educators from all backgrounds, so that they may come together to offer wider support to practitioners, to lobby and advocate for the profession as a whole and to ensure that smaller professions are not left behind in the move to improve standards of teaching and learning throughout the healthcare sector as a whole.

A common educational language that would allow wider conversations about healthcare teaching and learning to take place between professions on a clear and equal footing.

These basic common desiderata are what will eventually supply the springboard for truly interprofessional education across the entire healthcare education continuum.

AFTERWORD: The Future of Interprofessional Education

In this book we have argued that basic understandings of healthcare education may not be taken for granted, and that each profession has its own practices, language and understandings that add further barriers and challenges to the already complex field of interprofessional education. We have argued that truly interprofessional education can never be built effectively on ground that is not level – where each profession not only holds to its own understanding of good educational practice but is unable or unwilling to trust that this understanding is shared by other professions.

We have shown how a consensus around what all healthcare educators do and value must be built from the ground up, with as wide and open a discussion as possible, allowing each profession to value and articulate not only what is good about its own traditions but to recognise what it shares with other professions and appreciate and respect those areas that are unique and different.

The HEVA framework belongs to no one profession, and consequently it belongs to all. This is a vital step in opening out the conversation about how good healthcare education can become excellent, and how excellent educators can be recognised, supported, developed, recruited and retained throughout the health service.

We realise that the HEVA framework is just a small step towards a more equal and inclusive approach to healthcare education, but now that a basic understanding has been achieved, it is time to capitalise upon it, and to move on to the next phase. We would now like to throw down four major challenges for the field of healthcare education as a whole.

The first is to establish what generic skills are shared by all healthcare educators as they progress through their careers. This is a vital prerequisite if we are to introduce more effective training, career planning, recruitment and a levelling up of the place of education with respect to service delivery, research and management across the healthcare sector.

The second is to identify those additional skills and values which are specific to effective interprofessional educators, regardless of original professional background. The HEVA study has already given us some indication that these may involve particular values and complex skills which have not yet been explored in depth.

There is a third challenge, which the professions themselves may wish to take up: that of identifying if there are skills and values that are unique to certain professions' educators, or whether healthcare education skills and values are generic and the only difference is the subject matter to be taught. We are not in a position to hypothesise; this is a question for those professions themselves to resolve if they can.

The final challenge is the one we laid down at the start of this book – the need for improved collaboration between health professions education organisations. While people of goodwill within education providers, professional associations, learned societies, commissioners and regulators everywhere agree that there is a desperate need for a more combined and coherent approach to the preparation of future generations of healthcare professionals, good intentions and piecemeal approaches will not of themselves bring about the changes that are so earnestly desired. We have shown through our work in this book that it is possible to distil a common basic understanding of the work and values of all healthcare educators out of the current complex soup of professional guidance. We have indicated ways in which this shared understanding can usefully be extended and further developed. It is now time for professional organisations themselves to work together on this broadening foundation of consensus to develop the unified structures and systems that are necessary, such as deliberate and planned collaboration with cross-sector aims in view, mutual recognition of expertise and experience between individual practitioners, sharing of resources, joint conferences and learning opportunities, the development of genuinely interprofessional initiatives and the improved high-level influence that would come from speaking as a unified profession of healthcare educators. The creation of a truly interprofessional federation of healthcare education organisations around shared values and activities is one step closer. The mission of such a federation is now obvious; it is to mobilise all healthcare professions to collaborate on the improvement of recognition, conditions, training and career pathways for all healthcare educators, regardless of role, background or primary profession. Properly supported and recognised, it is these healthcare education professionals who will respond to the changing healthcare environment to bring about the improvements in interprofessional healthcare education that are so necessary to the formation of effective teams in clinical practice. In this way they will continue to deliver the primary mandate entrusted to healthcare educators for millennia – guiding and developing the next generation of clinicians to provide excellent patient care.

References

Academy for Healthcare Science. (2018). *AHCS standards of education and training for MSC undergraduate and postgraduate programmes*. Retrieved from https://www.ahcs.ac.uk/education-training/standards/

Academy of Medical Educators. (2014). *Professional standards for medical, dental and veterinary educators*. Retrieved from https://www.medicaleducators.org/Professional-Standards

Academy of Medical Royal Colleges (AoMRC). (2009). *Common competences framework for doctors*. Retrieved from https://www.aomrc.org.uk/wp-content/uploads/2018/03/CCFD-August-2009-1.pdf

Academy of Medical Royal Colleges (AoMRC) et al. (2017). *Joint professions' statement*. 2017. Retrieved from http://www.aomrc.org.uk/wp-content/uploads/2017/10/JOINT-PROFESSIONS-STATEMENT-111018.pdf

Academy of Medical Sciences. (2010). *Redressing the balance: the status and valuation of teaching in academic careers in the biomedical sciences*. Retrieved from https://acmedsci.ac.uk/file-download/35943-53b159424f36e.pdf

Accreditation of Interprofessional Health Education (AIPHE). (2014) *Principles and practices for integrating interprofessional education into the accreditation standards for six health professions in Canada*. Retrieved from https://casn.ca/wp-content/uploads/2014/12/AIPHEPrinciplesandPracticesGuidev2EN.pdf (accessed 28 May 2020)

Aguayo Gonzalez, M. P., & Monereo, C. (2012). The nurse teacher. Construction of a new professional identity. *Investigación y Educación en Enfermería*,

30(3). Retrieved from https://revistas.udea.edu.co/index.php/iee/article/view/11424

Albert M, Hodges B, & Regehr G. (2007). Research in medical education: Balancing service and science. *Advances in Health Sciences Education, 12,* 103–115.

Amorosa, J. M. H., Mellman, L. A., & Graham, M. J. (2011). Medical students as teachers: How preclinical teaching opportunities can create an early awareness of the role of physician as teacher. *Medical Teacher, 33*(2), 137–144. doi: https://doi.org/10.3109/0142159X.2010.531154

Archer, S., Hull, L., Soukup, T., Mayer, E., Athanasiou, T., Sevdalis, N., & Darzi, A. (2017). Development of a theoretical framework of factors affecting patient safety incident reporting: A theoretical review of the literature. *BMJ open, 7*(12), e017155–e017155. doi: https://doi.org/10.1136/bmjopen-2017-017155

Argyris, C. (1992). *On organisational learning.* Oxford: Blackwell Publishers Ltd.

Association for the Study of Medical Education (ASME). (2017). *Proposed federation of healthcare education report.* Retrieved from https://www.asme.org.uk/images/Report_on_Federation_Consultation_JB__JB-W_171113.pdf

Association for Medical Education in Europe The. (2011). *AMEE charter for medical educators.* Retrieved from https://amee.org/what-is-amee/an-amee-charter-for-medical-educators

Association for Simulated Practice in Healthcare The (ASPiH). (2016). *Simulation-based Education in Healthcare Standards Framework.* Retrieved from http://aspih.org.uk/wp-content/uploads/2017/07/standards-framework.pdf

Association of Child Psychotherapists, The. (2016). *Quality assurance framework for the training of child psychotherapists.* Retrieved from https://childpsychotherapy.org.uk/sites/default/files/documents/The%20Association%20of%20Child%20Psychotherapists%20-%20Quality%20Assurance%20Framework%20for%20the%20Training%20of%20Child%20Psychotherapists%20%28January%202016%29.pdf

Austerberry, H., & Newman, M. (2013). *Review of qualifications and training for clinical educators in the healthcare professions.* Retrieved from https://faculty.londondeanery.ac.uk/other-resources/review-of-qualifications-and-training-for-clinical-teachers-in-the-healthcare-professions-4

Australian Nurse Teachers' Society, The. (2010). *Australian nurse teacher professional practice standards.* Retrieved from https://www.ants.org.au/ants/mod/resource/view.php?id=600

Baerg, K., Lake, D., & Paslawski, T. (2012). Survey of interprofessional collaboration learning needs and training interest in health professionals, teachers, and students: An exploratory study. *Journal of Research in Interprofessional Practice and Education, 2*(2), 187–203. doi: http://dx.doi.org/10.22230/jripe.2012v2n2a47

Barleycorn, D., & Lee, G. A. (2018). How effective is trauma simulation as an educational process for healthcare providers within the trauma networks? A systematic review. *International Emergency Nursing, 40*, 37–45. doi: https://doi.org/10.1016/j.ienj.2018.03.007

Barr, H. (2002). *Interprofessional education: Today, yesterday and tomorrow.* In UK centre for the advancement of interprofessional education (Ed.). York: Learning and Teaching Support Network (subsequently Advance HE).

Barr, H., Ford, J., Gray, R., Helme, M., Hutchings, M., Low, H., Machin, A. & Reeves, S. (2017). *CAIPE interprofessional education guidelines.* Retrieved from https://www.caipe.org/resources/publications/caipe-publications/caipe-2017-interprofessional-education-guidelines-barr-h-ford-j-gray-r-helme-m-hutchings-m-low-h-machin-reeves-s

Bartle E, & Thistlethwaite J. (2014). Becoming a medical educator: Motivation, socialisation and navigation. *BMC Medical Education, 14*(1), 1–9.

Birks, Y., Harrison, R., Bosanquet, K., Hall, J., Harden, M., Entwistle, V., Watt, I., Walsh, P., Ronaldson, S., Roberts, D., & Adamson, J. (2014). An exploration of the implementation of open disclosure of adverse events in the UK: A scoping review and qualitative exploration. *Health Services and Delivery Research, 2*(20).

Bittner N. P., & Bechtel C. F. (2017). Identifying and describing nurse faculty workload issues: A looming faculty shortage. *Nursing Education Perspectives, 38*(4), 171–176.

Bleakley, A., Bligh, J., & Browne, J. (2011). *Medical education for the future: Identity, power and location.* Dordrecht: Springer.

British Association of Social Workers, The. (2018). *BASW Accreditation scheme for providers of continuing professional development for social workers: overview guide.* Retrieved from https://www.basw.co.uk/resources/basw-accreditation-scheme-overview-guide

British Dietetic Association, The. (2013). *A Curriculum Framework for the pre-registration education and training of dietitians.* Retrieved from https://www.bda.uk.com/practice-and-education/education/pre-registration.html

British Medical Association. (2006). *Doctors as teachers.* Retrieved from https://warwick.ac.uk/fac/sci/med/study/ugr/mbchb/societies/slime/products/teaching/doctors_as_teachers_bma_sept_06.pdf

Browne, J., Webb, K., & Bullock, A. (2018). Making the leap to medical education: A qualitative study of medical educators' experiences. *Medical Education, 52*, 216–226. doi: https://doi.org/10.1111/medu.13470

Browne, J. (2021). The role of professional bodies in health professions education. In D. Nestel, G. Reedy, L. McKenna, & S. Gough (Eds.), *Clinical education for the health professions.* Dordrecht: Springer.

Burgess, A., Kalman, E., Haq, I., Leaver, A., Roberts, C., & Bleasel, J. (2020). Interprofessional team-based learning (TBL): How do students engage?

BMC Medical Education, 20(1), 118. doi: https://doi.org/10.1186/s12909-020-02024-5

Burton, S., Boschmans, S.-A., & Hoelson, C. (2013). Self-perceived professional identity of pharmacy educators in South Africa. *American Journal of Pharmaceutical Education, 77*(10), 210. doi: https://doi.org/10.5688/ajpe7710210

Cantillon P., Dornan T., & De Grave W. (2019). Becoming a clinical teacher: Identity formation in context. *Academic Medicine, 94*(10), 1610–1618.

Carifio J., & Perla R. (2008). Resolving the 50-year debate around using and misusing Likert scales. *Medical Education, 42*(12), 1150–1152.

Chadaga, A. R., Villines, D., & Krikorian, A. (2016). Bullying in the American graduate medical education system: A national cross-sectional survey. *PloS One, 11*(3), e0150246–e0150246. doi: https://doi.org/10.1371/journal.pone.0150246

Chartered Society of Physiotherapy. (2014). *Accreditation of clinical educators scheme*. Retrieved from http://www.csp.org.uk/sites/files/csp/csp_clinical_ed_ace_041.htm#documentation

Chuenjitwongsa S. (2017). *How to conduct a Delphi study*. Wales Deanery. Retrieved from https://meded.walesdeanery.org/sites/default/files/how_to_conduct_a_delphistudy.pdf

Christensen, L.S. & Simmons, L.E. (2020). *The Scope of Practice for Academic Nurse Educators and Academic Clinical Nurse Educators (3rd ed.)*. Washington, DC: National League for Nursing.

Clarke, C., Kane, D., Rajacich, D., & Lafreniere, K. (2012). Bullying in undergraduate clinical nursing education. *Journal of Nursing Education, 51*(5), 269–276.

College of Operating Department Practitioners. *Standards, recommendations and guidance for mentors and practice placements*. Retrieved from https://www.unison.org.uk/content/uploads/2017/11/CODP-Standards-recommendations-and-guidance-for-mentors-and-practice-placements.pdf

College of Paramedics, The. (2017). *Practice educator guidance handbook*. Bridgwater, UK: College of Paramedics.

College of Social Work, The. (2013). *Practice educator professional standards for social work*. Retrieved from https://www.basw.co.uk/resources/practice-educator-professional-standards-social-work-tcsw-archive

Committee of Postgraduate Dental Deans and Directors UK (COPDEND). (2013). *Standards for dental educators*. Retrieved from https://www.copdend.org/wp-content/uploads/2018/08/Guidelines-for-Dental-Educators-.pdf#:~:text=In%20presenting%20these%20Standards%2C%20COPDEND,educational%20content%20for%20dental%20educators.

Committee on Standards in Public Life. (1995). *Standards in Public Life (The Nolan Report)*. London: Her Majesty's Stationery Office.

Commission on Education and Training for Patient Safety. (2016). *Improving safety through education and training*. Retrieved from https://www.hee.nhs

.uk/sites/default/files/documents/Improving%20safety%20through%20education%20and%20training.pdf

Crosby, J., & Harden, R. M. (2000). AMEE Guide No 20: The good teacher is more than a lecturer – The twelve roles of the teacher. *Medical Teacher, 22*(4), 334–347. doi: https://doi.org/10.1080/014215900409429

Darbishire, P., Isaacs, A. N., & Miller, M. L. (2020). Faculty burnout in pharmacy education. *American Journal of Pharmaceutical Education*, ajpe7925. doi: https://doi.org/10.5688/ajpe7925

Dekker, S. (2013). *Second victim: Error, guilt, trauma, and resilience.* Boca Raton, FL: CRC Press.

Dahlstrom, J., Dorai-Raj, A., McGill, D., Owen, C., Tymms, K., & Watson, D. A. R. (2005). What motivates senior clinicians to teach medical students? *BMC Medical Education, 5*, 27–27. doi: https://doi.org/10.1186/1472-6920-5-27

Delbecq A. L., van de Ven A. H., & Gustafson D. H. (1986). *Group techniques for program planning: A guide to nominal group and Delphi processes.* Middleton WI: Green Briar Press.

de Villiers M. R., de Villiers P. J., & Kent A. P. (2005). The Delphi technique in health sciences education research. *Medical Teacher, 27*(7), 639–643.

Diamond I. R. et al. (2014). Defining consensus: A systematic review recommends methodologic criteria for reporting of Delphi studies. *Journal of Clinical Epidemiology, 67*(4), 401–409

Draugalis, J. R., DiPiro, J. T., Zeolla, M. M., & Schwinghammer, T. L. (2006). A career in academic pharmacy: opportunities, challenges, and rewards. *American Journal of Pharmaceutical Education, 70*(1), 17–17. doi: https://doi.org/10.5688/aj700117

Dybowski, C., & Harendza, S. (2014). "Teaching Is Like Nightshifts …": A focus group study on the teaching motivations of clinicians. *Teaching and Learning in Medicine, 26*(4), 393–400. doi: https://doi.org/10.1080/10401334.2014.910467

Engeström, Y. (1987). *Learning by expanding: An activity-theoretical approach to development research.* Helsinki: Orienta-Konsultit.

Faculty of Medical Leadership and Management. *Leadership and management standards for medical professionals. (2nd edition).* Retrieved from: https://www.fmlm.ac.uk/individual-standards

Foronda, C., MacWilliams, B., & McArthur, E. (2016). Interprofessional communication in healthcare: An integrative review. *Nurse Education in Practice, 19*, 36–40. doi: https://doi.org/10.1016/j.nepr.2016.04.005

Francis, R. (2013). *Report of the Mid Staffordshire NHS Trust public inquiry.* Retrieved from https://www.gov.uk/government/publications/report-of-the-mid-staffordshire-nhs-foundation-trust-public-inquiry

Frank, J.R., Snell, L., & Sherbino, J. (Eds.) (2015). *CanMEDS 2015 Physician competency framework.* Ottawa: Royal College of Physicians and Surgeons of Canada.

Freeth, D. (2010). Interprofessional education. In T. Swanwick (Ed.), *Understanding medical education: Evidence, theory and practice* (pp. 53–68). Oxford: Blackwell.

Frenk J., Chen L., Bhutta Z. A., Cohen J., Crisp N., Evans T., Fineberg H., Garcia P., Ke Y., Kelley P., & Kistnasamy B. (2010). Health professionals for a new century: Transforming education to strengthen health systems in an interdependent world. *The Lancet, 376*(9756), 1923–1958.

Fullerton, L., Oglesbee, S., Weiss, S. J., Ernst, A. A., & Mesic, V. (2019). Assessing the prevalence and predictors of bullying among emergency medical service providers. *Prehospital Emergency Care, 23*(1), 9–14. doi: https://doi.org/10.1080/10903127.2018.1470208

Gandhi, T. K., Berwick, D. M., & Shojania, K. G. (2016). Patient safety at the crossroads. *JAMA, 315*(17), 1829–1830. doi: https://doi.org/10.1001/jama.2016.1759

General Medical Council. *Recognising and approving trainers: the implementation plan.* Retrieved from https://www.gmc-uk.org/education/standards-guidance-and-curricula/position-statements/recognising-and-approving-trainers-implementation-plan

General Medical Council. *Promoting excellence: standards for medical education and training.* Retrieved from https://www.gmc-uk.org/education/standards-guidance-and-curricula/standards-and-outcomes/promoting-excellence

Government of South Australia. *Medical education and training principles.* Retrieved from https://www.sahealth.sa.gov.au/wps/wcm/connect/c571fa1b-488d-4096-8e28-6575e92c768a/18105.1+SA+Met_Strategic+Priority+doc_2018+Update_WEB+2.pdf?MOD=AJPERES&CACHEID=ROOTWORKSPACE-c571fa1b-488d-4096-8e28-6575e92c768a-n5iq2Td

Gunderman, R. (2006). *Achieving excellence in medical education.* London: Springer-Verlag Limited.

Hafferty, F. W., & O'Donnell, J. F. (2014). *The hidden curriculum in health professional education.* Hanover, NH: Dartmouth College Press.

Hammick, M., Freeth, D., Koppel, I., Reeves, S., & Barr, H. (2007). A best evidence systematic review of interprofessional education: BEME Guide no. 9. *Medical Teacher, 29*(8), 735–751. doi: https://doi.org/10.1080/01421590701682576

Hand J. S. (2006) Identification of competencies for effective dental faculty. *Journal of Dental Education 70*(9), 937–947.

Health and Care Professions Council. *Standards of education and training.* Retrieved from https://www.hcpc-uk.org/standards/standards-relevant-to-education-and-training/set/

Health Education North West. (2014a). *Clinical supervision in Health Education North West.* Retrieved from https://www.nwpgmd.nhs.uk/sites/default/files/CS%20in%20HENW%20-%20Overview%202014_1.pdf

Health Education North West. (2014b). *Educational supervision in Health Education North West*. Retrieved from https://www.bfwh.nhs.uk/onehr/wp-content/uploads/2016/10/ES-in-HENW-Overview-2014.pdf

Health Foundation, The. (2011). *Levels of harm in healthcare*. Retrieved from London: https://www.health.org.uk/publications/levels-of-harm

Health Professions Network Nursing and Midwifery Office. (2010). *Framework for action on interprofessional education and collaborative practice* (World Health Organisation Ed.). Geneva: World Health Organisation.

Higher Education Academy, The. (2011). *The UK professional standards framework for teaching and supporting learning in higher education*. York: HEA.

Holt J., Coates C., Cotterill D., Eastburn S., Laxton J., Mistry H., & Young C. (2010). Identifying common competences in health and social care: An example of multi-institutional and inter-professional working. *Nurse Education Today*, 30(3), 264–270.

Hu, W. C. Y., Thistlethwaite, J. E., Weller, J., Gallego, G., Monteith, J., & McColl, G. J. (2015). 'It was serendipity': A qualitative study of academic careers in medical education. *Medical Education, 49*(11), 1124–1136. doi: https://doi.org/10.1111/medu.12822

Institute of Medicine Committee on Quality of Health Care, Kohn, L. T., Corrigan, J. M., & Donaldson, M. S. (2000). *To err is human: Building a safer health system*. Washington (DC): National Academies Press.

International Confederation of Midwives. *Global standards for midwifery education*. Retrieved from https://www.internationalmidwives.org/assets/files/general-files/2018/04/icm-standards-guidelines_ammended2013.pdf

Interprofessional Education Collaborative. *Core competencies for interprofessional collaborative practice: 2016 update*. Retrieved from https://nebula.wsimg.com/2f68a39520b03336b41038c370497473?AccessKeyId=DC06780E69ED19E2B3A5&disposition=0&alloworigin=1

Irish Network of Medical Educators. *Charter of best practice in medicine, dentistry, and pharmacy*. Cork: INMED. Retrieved from https://www.inhed.ie/wp-content/uploads/2018/05/INMED-Charter-of-Best-Practice.pdf

Jones J., & Hunter D. (1995). Qualitative research: Consensus methods for medical and health services research. *British Medical Journal*, 311, 376–380.

Kapur, N., Parand, A., Soukup, T., Reader, T., & Sevdalis, N. (2015). Aviation and healthcare: A comparative review with implications for patient safety. *JRSM open, 7*(1). doi: https://doi.org/10.1177/2054270415616548

King, D. B., O'Rourke, N., & DeLongis, A. (2014). Social media recruitment and online data collection: A beginner's guide and best practices for accessing low-prevalence and hard-to-reach populations. *Canadian Psychology/Psychologie canadienne, 55*(4), 240–249. https://doi.org/10.1037/a0038087

Kirkup, W. (2015). *The report of the Morecambe Bay investigation*. Retrieved from https://assets.publishing.service.gov.uk/government/uploads/system/uploads/attachment_data/file/408480/47487_MBI_Accessible_v0.1.pdf

Knapp, K., Shane, P., Sasaki-Hill, D., Yoshizuka, K., Chan, P., & Vo, T. (2014). Bullying in the clinical training of pharmacy students. *American Journal of Pharmaceutical Education, 78*(6), 117. doi: https://doi.org/10.5688/ajpe786117

Lark, M. E., Kirkpatrick, K., & Chung, K. C. (2018). Patient safety movement: History and future directions. *The Journal of Hand Surgery, 43*(2), 174–178. doi: https://doi.org/10.1016/j.jhsa.2017.11.006

Leggate, M., & Russell, E. (2002). Attitudes and trends of primary care dentists to continuing professional development: A report from the Scottish dental practitioners survey 2000. *British Dental Journal, 193*(8), 465–469. doi: https://doi.org/10.1038/sj.bdj.4801598

Lingard, L. (2012). Rethinking competence in the context of teamwork. In B. Hodges & L. Lingard (Eds.), *The question of competence: Reconsidering medical education in the twenty-first century* (pp. 42–69). Ithaca, NY: Cornell University Press.

Lingard, L., Sue-Chue-Lam, C., Tait, G. R., Bates, J., Shadd, J., Schulz, V., . . . For the Heart Failure/Palliative Care Teamwork Research Group. (2017). Pulling together and pulling apart: influences of convergence and divergence on distributed healthcare teams. *Advances in Health Sciences Education, 22*(5), 1085–1099. doi: https://doi.org/10.1007/s10459-016-9741-2

McCrann, S., Flitcroft, I., & Loughman, J. (2020). Is optometry ready for myopia control? Education and other barriers to the treatment of myopia [version 2; peer review: 1 approved with reservations]. *HRB Open Research, 2*(30). doi: https://doi.org/10.12688/hrbopenres.12954.2

McFadden Kathleen, L., Stock Gregory, N., & Gowen Charles, R. (2006). Implementation of patient safety initiatives in US hospitals. *International Journal of Operations & Production Management, 26*(3), 326–347. doi: https://doi.org/10.1108/01443570610651052

Mladenovic, J., & Tilden, V. P. (2017). Strategies for overcoming barriers to IPE at a health sciences university. *Journal of Interprofessional Education & Practice, 8*, 10–13. doi: https://doi.org/10.1016/j.xjep.2017.05.002

Molloy, E., & Bearman, M. (2019). Embracing the tension between vulnerability and credibility: 'Intellectual candour' in health professions education. *Medical Education, 53*(1), 32–41. doi: https://doi.org/10.1111/medu.13649

Monrouxe, L. V., Rees, C. E., Dennis, I., & Wells, S. E. (2015). Professionalism dilemmas, moral distress and the healthcare student: Insights from two online UK-wide questionnaire studies. *BMJ Open, 5*(5), e007518. doi: https://doi.org/10.1136/bmjopen-2014-007518

Nancarrow, S. A., & Borthwick, A. M. (2005). Dynamic professional boundaries in the healthcare workforce. *Sociology of Health & Illness, 27*(7), 897–919

National Centre for Biotechnology Information. *US National Library of Medicine Catalog*. Retrieved from https://www.ncbi.nlm.nih.gov/nlmcatalog

National School of Healthcare Science. *NHS scientist training programme helpbook for training centres*. Retrieved from https://nshcs.hee.nhs.uk/news/stp-helpbook-for-training-centres/

Neese, R. (2003). A transformational journey from clinician to educator. *The Journal of Continuing Education in Nursing, 36*(4), 258–262. doi: https://doi.org/10.3928/0022-0124-20031101-08

NHS England, Public Health England, Health Education England, Monitor, Care Quality Commission, NHS Trust Development Authority *Five Year Forward View*. Retrieved from http://www.england.nhs.uk/wp-content/uploads/2014/10/5yfv-web.pdf

NHS England. (2017). *Next steps on the NHS five year forward view*. Retrieved from https://www.england.nhs.uk/five-year-forward-view/next-steps-on-the-nhs-five-year-forward-view/primary-care/

NHS Long-Term Plan (2019). Retrieved from https://www.longtermplan.nhs.uk/

Norman G. (2010), Likert scales, levels of measurement and the "laws" of statistics. *Advances in Health Sciences Education, 15*(5), 625–632.

Nursing and Midwifery Board of Ireland. *Midwife registration programme standards and requirements*. Retrieved from https://www.nmbi.ie/Education/Standards-and-Requirements

Nursing and Midwifery Council, The. *Standards to support learning and assessment in practice*. Retrieved from https://www.nmc.org.uk/standards-for-education-and-training/standards-to-support-learning-and-assessment-in-practice/

Parrott L., Lee A., & Markless S. (2017). The perceptions of dental practitioners of their role as clinical teachers in a UK outreach dental clinic. *British Dental Journal, 222*, 107–112.

Powell C. (2003). The Delphi technique: Myths and realities. *Journal of Advanced Nursing, 41*(4), 376–382.

Powell, M. (2020). The duty of candour and the NHS agenda. *International Journal of Health Governance, [Published ahead of print]*. doi: https://doi-org.abc.cardiff.ac.uk/10.1108/IJHG-01-2020-0005

QSR International Pty Ltd. (2018). NVivo (Version 12). Retrieved from https://www.qsrinternational.com/nvivo-qualitative-data-analysis-software/home

Reason, J. (2000). Human error: Models and management. *BMJ (Clinical Research Ed.), 320*(7237), 768–770. doi: https://doi.org/10.1136/bmj.320.7237.768

Riveros-Perez, E., & Rodriguez-Diaz, J. (2017). The journey from clinician to undergraduate medical educator involves four patterns of transformation. *Advances in Medical Education and Practice, 9*, 7–15. doi: https://doi.org/10.2147/AMEP.S146384

Royal College of Occupational Therapists, The (2019). *Learning and development standards for pre-registration education*. Retrieved from https://www

.rcot.co.uk/practice-resources/rcot-publications/learning-and-development-standards-pre-registration-education

Royal College of Surgeons of Edinburgh, The. *Standards for surgical trainers.* Retrieved from https://fst.rcsed.ac.uk/media/15968/standards-for-surgical-trainers-version-2.pdf

Royal Pharmaceutical Society. (2015). *Tutor guidance.* Retrieved from https://www.rpharms.com/Portals/0/RPS%20document%20library/Open%20access/Development/Tutor/tutor-guidance-2015.pdf

Royal Pharmaceutical Society. (Undated) *Draft standards for RPS tutors (supervisors).* (Retrieved from https://www.rpharms.com/Portals/0/RPS%20document%20library/Open%20access/Development/Tutor/Draft%20Standards%20for%20RPS%20Tutors%20(Supervisors).pdf?ver=2017-04-07-131727-220

Royal Pharmaceutical Society. (Undated). *RPS draft standards for workplace facilitators (supervisors).* Retrieved from https://www.rpharms.com/Portals/0/RPS%20document%20library/Open%20access/Development/Tutor/Draft%20Standards%20for%20Workplace%20Facilitators%20%28Supervisors%29.pdf

Royal Pharmaceutical Society. (2013). *Advanced pharmacy framework (APF).* Retrieved from https://www.rpharms.com/Portals/0/RPS%20document%20library/Open%20access/Frameworks/RPS%20Advanced%20Pharmacy%20Framework.pdf

Russell, S., & Foulkes, I. (2019). Embedding a positive research culture that fosters innovation. *Nature Reviews Cancer, 19*(5), 241–242. doi: https://doi.org/10.1038/s41568-019-0127-7

Sabel, E., Archer, J., & on behalf of the Early Careers Working Group at the Academy of Medical Educators. (2014). "Medical education is the ugly duckling of the medical world" and other challenges to medical educators' identity construction: A qualitative study. *Academic Medicine, 89*(11). Retrieved from https://journals.lww.com/academicmedicine/Fulltext/2014/11000/_Medical_Education_Is_the_Ugly_Duckling_of_the.25.aspx

Salas, E., Sims, D. E., & Burke, C. S. (2005). Is there a 'big five' in teamwork? *Small Group Research, 36*(5), 555–599. doi: https://doi.org/10.1177/1046496405277134

Schoening, A. (2013). From bedside to classroom: The nurse educator transition model. *Nursing Education Perspectives, 34*(3), 167–172. Retrieved from https://journals.lww.com/neponline/Fulltext/2013/05000/From_Bedside_to_Classroom_The_Nurse_Educator.7.aspx

Secretary of State for Health. (2015). *Culture change: Applying the lessons of the Francis Inquiries.* Retrieved from https://assets.publishing.service.gov.uk/government/uploads/system/uploads/attachment_data/file/403010/culture-change-nhs.pdf

Sethi, A., Ajjawi, R., McAleer, S., & Schofield, S. (2017). Exploring the tensions of being and becoming a medical educator. *BMC Medical Education, 17*(1), 62. doi: https://doi.org/10.1186/s12909-017-0894-3

Sevens, T.J., & Reeves, P. J. (2019). Professional protectionism: A barrier to employing a sonographer graduate? *Radiography, 25*(1), 77–82.

Social Care Workers Registration Board (CORU). *Criteria for Education and Training Programmes – Guidelines for Programme Providers.* Retrieved from https://www.coru.ie/files-education/scwrb-criteria-for-education-and-training-programmes.pdf

Spencer, J. (2003). Learning and teaching in the clinical environment. *BMJ (Clinical Research Ed.), 326*(7389), 591–594. doi: https://doi.org/10.1136/bmj.326.7389.591

Steinert, Y. (2005). Learning together to teach together: Interprofessional education and faculty development. *Journal of Interprofessional Care, 19*(sup1), 60–75. doi: https://doi.org/10.1080/13561820500081778

Steinert, Y., O'Sullivan, P. S., & Irby, D. M. (2019). Strengthening teachers' professional identities through faculty development. *Acad Med, 94*(7), 963–968. doi: https://doi.org/10.1097/acm.0000000000002695

Sutcliffe, K. M., Lewton, E., & Rosenthal, M. M. (2004). Communication failures: An insidious contributor to medical mishaps. *Academic Medicine, 79*(2), 186–194. Retrieved from https://journals.lww.com/academicmedicine/Fulltext/2004/02000/Communication_Failures__An_Insidious_Contributor.19.aspx

Thistlethwaite, J. E., Forman, D., Matthews, L. R., Rogers, G. D., Steketee, C., & Yassine, T. (2014). Competencies and frameworks in interprofessional education: A comparative analysis. *Academic Medicine, 89*(6), 869–875.

Turner, T. L., Palazzi, D. L., & Ward, M. A. 2008. *The clinician educator's handbook.* Houston: Baylor College of Medicine. Retrieved from https://media.bcm.edu/documents/2014/84/clinicianedhandbook.pdf

Uhling, P. N., Doll, J., Brandon, K., Goodman, C., Medado-Ramirez, J., Barnes, M. A., Dolansky, M. A., Ratcliffe, T. A., Kornsawad, K., Raboin, W. E., & Hitzeman, M. (2018). Interprofessional practice and education in clinical learning environments: Frontlines perspective. *Academic Medicine, 93*(10), 1441–1444.

UK Council for Psychotherapy. *UKCP standards of education and training.* Retrieved from https://www.psychotherapy.org.uk/wp-content/uploads/2017/02/Standards-of-Education-and-Training-2017SETs.pdf

Van Der Vleuten, C. P. M., & Schuwirth, L. W. T. (2005). Assessing professional competence: From methods to programmes. *Medical Education, 39*(3), 309–317. doi: https://doi.org/10.1111/j.1365-2929.2005.02094.x

Vincent, C., Taylor-Adams, S., & Stanhope, N. (1998). Framework for analysing risk and safety in clinical medicine. *BMJ, 316*(7138), 1154–1157. doi: https://doi.org/10.1136/bmj.316.7138.1154

Walsh, A., Antao, V., Bethune, C., Cameron, S., Cavett, T., Clavet, D., Dove, M., & Koppula, S. (2015). *Fundamental teaching activities in family medicine: A framework for faculty development.* Mississauga, ON: College of Family Physicians of Canada. Retrieved from https://portal.cfpc.ca/resourcesdocs/uploadedFiles/Education/_PDFs/FTA_GUIDE_TM_ENG_Apr15_REV.pdf

Weller, J. (2012). Shedding new light on tribalism in health care. *Medical Education*, 46, 134–136. doi: https://doi.org/10.1111/j.1365-2923.2011.04178.x

West M., Armit K., Loewethal L., et al. (2015). *Leadership and leadership development in health care: The evidence base*. Retrieved from https://www.kingsfund.org.uk/publications/leadership-and-leadership-development-health-care

World Federation for Medical Education. (2015). *Basic medical education: WFME global standards for quality improvement*. WFME: Ferney-Voltaire and Copenhagen.

World Federation of Occupational Therapists. (2016). *Minimum standards for the education of occupational therapists*. Retrieved from https://www.wfot.org/assets/resources/COPYRIGHTED-World-Federation-of-Occupational-Therapists-Minimum-Standards-for-the-Education-of-Occupational-Therapists-2016a.pdf

World Health Organisation. (2014). *Midwifery educator core competencies*. Retrieved from https://www.who.int/hrh/nursing_midwifery/midwifery_educator_core_competencies.pdf?ua=1

World Health Organisation. (2016). *Nurse educator core competencies*. Retrieved from https://apps.who.int/iris/bitstream/handle/10665/258713/9789241549622-eng.pdf;jsessionid=B44ED17ECA84A88F6995995A22310A32?sequence=1

World Health Organisation. (2017). *Patient safety: Making health care safer*. Retrieved from Geneva: https://apps.who.int/iris/handle/10665/255507

Wu, A. W. (2000). Medical error: The second victim: The doctor who makes the mistake needs help too. *BMJ: British Medical Journal*, 320(7237), 726–727. Retrieved from www.jstor.org/stable/25187393

Appendix 1: List of Standards Documents Analysed

Organisation	Reference	Key audience
Academy of Medical Royal Colleges	Academy of Medical Royal Colleges. *Common Competences Framework for Doctors*. Retrieved from London: https://www.aomrc.org.uk/wp-content/uploads/2018/03/CCFD-August-2009-1.pdf	Doctors
The Academy of Medical Sciences	Academy of Medical Sciences. (2010). *Redressing the balance: the status and valuation of teaching in academic careers in the biomedical sciences*. Retrieved from: https://acmedsci.ac.uk/file-download/35943-53b159424f36e.pdf	Biomedical Scientists
Academy for Healthcare Science (AHCS)	Academy for Healthcare Science (2018). *AHCS Standards of Education and Training for MSC Undergraduate and Postgraduate Programmes*. Retrieved from: https://www.ahcs.ac.uk/education-training/standards/	Multi-professional healthcare
Association for Medical Education in Europe (AMEE)	The Association for Medical Education in Europe (2011). *AMEE Charter for Medical Educators*. Retrieved from: https://amee.org/what-is-amee/an-amee-charter-for-medical-educators	Doctors

(Cont'd.)

Organisation	Reference	Key audience
The Australian Nurse Teachers' Society (ANTS)	The Australian Nurse Teachers' Society (2010). *Australian Nurse Teacher Professional Practice Standards*. Retrieved from: https://www.ants.org.au/ants/mod/resource/view.php?id=600	Nurses
Academy of Medical Educators (AoME)	Academy of Medical Educators (2014). *Professional Standards for Medical, Dental and Veterinary Educators* Retrieved from: https://www.medicaleducators.org/Professional-Standards	Doctors, dentists, vets
Association for Simulated Practice in Healthcare (ASPiH)	The Association for Simulated Practice in Healthcare (ASPiH) (2016). *Simulation-based Education in Healthcare Standards Framework*. Retrieved from: http://aspih.org.uk/wp-content/uploads/2017/07/standards-framework.pdf	Multi-professional healthcare
British Association of Social Workers (BASW)	The British Association of Social Workers (2018). *BASW Accreditation scheme for providers of continuing professional development for social workers: overview guide*. Retrieved from: https://www.basw.co.uk/resources/basw-accreditation-scheme-overview-guide	Social Work
BMA Board of Medical Education	British Medical Association (2006). *Doctors as teachers*. Retrieved from: https://warwick.ac.uk/fac/sci/med/study/ugr/mbchb/societies/slime/products/teaching/doctors_as_teachers_bma_sept_06.pdf	Doctors
British Dietetic Association	The British Dietetic Association (2013). *A Curriculum Framework for the pre-registration education and training of dietitians*. Retrieved from: https://www.bda.uk.com/practice-and-education/education/pre-registration.html	Dietitians
Centre for the Advancement of Interprofessional Education (CAIPE)	Barr, H Barr et al. (2017). *CAIPE Interprofessional Education Guidelines*. Retrieved from https://www.caipe.org/resources/publications/caipe-publications/caipe-2017-interprofessional-education-guidelines-barr-h-ford-j-gray-r-helme-m-hutchings-m-low-h-machin-reeves-s	Multi-professional healthcare
CanMEDS - Royal College of Physicians and Surgeons of Canada	Frank et al. CanMEDS (2015). *Physician Competency Framework*. Ottawa: Royal College of Physicians and Surgeons of Canada.	Doctors

Organisation	Reference	Key audience
Chartered Society of Physiotherapy	Chartered Society of Physiotherapy (2014). *Accreditation of Clinical Educators Scheme*. Retrieved from: http://www.csp.org.uk/sites/files/csp/csp_clinical_ed_ace_041.htm#documentation [last accessed 8/3/2018, subsequently withdrawn and archived].	Physiotherapists
The Clinician-Educator's Handbook	Turner et al. (2008). *The Clinician Educator's Handbook*. Houston: Baylor College of Medicine. Retrieved from: https://media.bcm.edu/documents/2014/84/clinicianedhandbook.pdf	Physician assistants
College of Operating Department Practitioners (CODP)	College of Operating Department Practitioners. *Standards, recommendations and guidance for mentors and practice placements*. Retrieved from: https://www.unison.org.uk/content/uploads/2017/11/CODP-Standards-recommendations-and-guidance-for-mentors-and-practice-placements.pdf	Doctors
The College of Family Physicians of Canada	Walsh et al. (2015). *Fundamental Teaching Activities in Family Medicine: A Framework for Faculty Development*. Mississauga, ON: College of Family Physicians of Canada. Retrieved from: https://portal.cfpc.ca/resourcesdocs/uploadedFiles/Education/_PDFs/FTA_GUIDE_TM_ENG_Apr15_REV.pdf	Doctors
Royal College of Occupational Therapists	Royal College of Occupational Therapists (2019). *Learning and development standards for pre-registration education*. Retrieved from: https://www.rcot.co.uk/practice-resources/rcot-publications/learning-and-development-standards-pre-registration-education	Occupational Therapists
College of Paramedics	College of Paramedics (2017). *Practice Educator Guidance Handbook*. Bridgwater, UK: College of Paramedics.	Paramedics
Committee of Postgraduate Dental Deans and Directors (COPDEND)	Committee of Postgraduate Dental Deans and Directors UK. (2013). *Standards for Dental Educators*. Retrieved from: https://www.copdend.org/wp-content/uploads/2018/08/Guidelines-for-Dental-Educators-.pdf#:~:text=In%20presenting%20these%20Standards%2C%20COPDEND,educational%20content%20for%20dental%20educators.	Dentists

(Cont'd.)

Organisation	Reference	Key audience
Social Care Workers Registration Board (CORU)	Social Care Workers Registration Board (CORU). *Criteria for Education and Training Programmes – Guidelines for Programme Providers.* Retrieved from: https://www.coru.ie/files-education/scwrb-criteria-for-education-and-training-programmes.pdf	Social Care Work
Faculty of Medical Leadership and Management (FMLM)	Faculty of Medical Leadership and Management. *Leadership and Management Standards for Medical Professionals.* (2nd edition) Retrieved from: https://www.fmlm.ac.uk/individual-standards	Doctors
General Medical Council (GMC)	General Medical Council. *Recognising and approving trainers: the implementation plan.* Retrieved from https://www.gmc-uk.org/education/standards-guidance-and-curricula/position-statements/recognising-and-approving-trainers-implementation-plan	Doctors
General Medical Council (GMC)	General Medical Council. *Promoting excellence: standards for medical education and training.* Retrieved from: https://www.gmc-uk.org/education/standards-guidance-and-curricula/standards-and-outcomes/promoting-excellence	Doctors
Health and Care Professions Council (HCPC)	Health and Care Professions Council. *Standards of Education and Training.* Retrieved from: https://www.hcpc-uk.org/standards/standards-relevant-to-education-and-training/set/	Multi-professional healthcare
Health Education England North West (HEE NW)	Health Education North West (2014a). *Clinical supervision in Health Education North West.* Retrieved from: https://www.nwpgmd.nhs.uk/sites/default/files/CS%20in%20HENW%20-%20Overview%202014_1.pdf Health Education North West (2014b). *Educational supervision in Health Education North West.* Retrieved from: https://www.bfwh.nhs.uk/onehr/wp-content/uploads/2016/10/ES-in-HENW-Overview-2014.pdf	Doctors
International Confederation of Midwives (ICM)	International Confederation of Midwives. *Global Standards for Midwifery Education.* Retrieved from: https://www.internationalmidwives.org/assets/files/general-files/2018/04/icm-standards-guidelines_ammended2013.pdf	Midwives

Appendix 1: List of Standards Documents Analysed   133

Organisation	Reference	Key audience
Irish Network of Medical Educators (INMED)	Irish Network of Medical Educators (2018). *Charter of Best Practice in Medicine, Dentistry, and Pharmacy*. Cork: INMED. Retrieved from: https://www.inhed.ie/wp-content/uploads/2018/05/INMED-Charter-of-Best-Practice.pdf (Note: since 2019, the organisation has become known as INHED, The Irish Network of Healthcare Educators.)	Doctors, dentists, pharmacists
Interprofessional Education Collaborative (IPEC)	Interprofessional Education Collaborative. *Core competencies for interprofessional collaborative practice: 2016 update*. Retrieved from: https://nebula.wsimg.com/2f68a39520b03336b41038c370497473?AccessKeyId=DC06780E69ED19E2B3A5&disposition=0&alloworigin=1	Multi-professional healthcare
National School of Healthcare Science (NSchHS)	National School of Healthcare Science. *NHS Scientist Training Programme Helpbook for Training Centres*. Retrieved from: https://nshcs.hee.nhs.uk/news/stp-helpbook-for-training-centres/	Biomedical Scientists
National League for Nursing (NLN)	Christensen, L..S and Simmons, L.E. (2020). *The Scope of Practice for Academic Nurse Educators and Academic Clinical Nurse Educators (3rd ed.)*. Washington, DC: National League for Nursing.)	Nurses
Nursing and Midwifery Board Ireland (NMBI)	Nursing and Midwifery Board of Ireland. *Midwife Registration Programme Standards and Requirements*. Retrieved from: https://www.nmbi.ie/Education/Standards-and-Requirements	Midwives
Nursing and Midwifery Council (NMC)	Nursing and Midwifery Council. *Standards to support learning and assessment in practice*. Retrieved from: https://www.nmc.org.uk/standards-for-education-and-training/standards-to-support-learning-and-assessment-in-practice/	Nurses
The College of Social Work	The College of Social Work (2013). *Practice Educator Professional Standards for Social Work*. https://www.basw.co.uk/resources/practice-educator-professional-standards-social-work-tcsw-archive	Social Work

(Cont'd.)

Organisation	Reference	Key audience
Royal College of Surgeons	The Royal College of Surgeons of Edinburgh. *Standards for Surgical Trainers*. Retrieved from: https://fst.rcsed.ac.uk/media/15968/standards-for-surgical-trainers-version-2.pdf	Doctors
Royal Pharmaceutical Society (RPS)	Royal Pharmaceutical Society. *Tutor Guidance*. Retrieved from: https://www.rpharms.com/Portals/0/RPS%20document%20library/Open%20access/Development/Tutor/tutor-guidance-2015.pdf	Pharmacists
	Royal Pharmaceutical Society. *Draft Standards for RPS Tutors (Supervisors)*. Retrieved from: https://www.rpharms.com/Portals/0/RPS%20document%20library/Open%20access/Development/Tutor/Draft%20Standards%20for%20RPS%20Tutors%20(Supervisors).pdf?ver=2017-04-07-131727-220	
	Royal Pharmaceutical Society. *RPS Draft Standards for Workplace Facilitators (Supervisors)*. Retrieved from: https://www.rpharms.com/Portals/0/RPS%20document%20library/Open%20access/Development/Tutor/Draft%20Standards%20for%20Workplace%20Facilitators%20%28Supervisors%29.pdf	
	Royal Pharmaceutical Society. *Advanced Pharmacy Framework (APF)*. Retrieved from: https://www.rpharms.com/Portals/0/RPS%20document%20library/Open%20access/Frameworks/RPS%20Advanced%20Pharmacy%20Framework.pdf	
Government of South Australia/ South Australian Medical Education and Training Education Committee	Government of South Australia. *Medical education and training principles*. Retrieved from: https://www.sahealth.sa.gov.au/wps/wcm/connect/c571fa1b-488d-4096-8e28-6575e92c768a/18105.1+SA+Met_Strategic+Priority+doc_2018+Update_WEB+2.pdf?MOD=AJPERES&CACHEID=ROOTWORKSPACE-c571fa1b-488d-4096-8e28-6575e92c768a-n5iq2Td	Doctors

Appendix 1: List of Standards Documents Analysed 135

Organisation	Reference	Key audience
The Association of Child Psychotherapists	The Association of Child Psychotherapists. *Quality Assurance Framework for the Training of Child Psychotherapists*. Retrieved from: https://childpsychotherapy.org.uk/sites/default/files/documents/The%20Association%20of%20Child%20Psychotherapists%20-%20Quality%20Assurance%20Framework%20for%20the%20Training%20of%20Child%20Psychotherapists%20%28January%202016%29.pdf.	Psychologists/ Psychotherapists
UK Council for Psychotherapy (UKCP)	UK Council for Psychotherapy. *UKCP Standards of Education and Training*. Retrieved from: Available at: https://www.psychotherapy.org.uk/wp-content/uploads/2017/02/Standards-of-Education-and-Training-2017SETs.pdf	Psychologists/ Psychotherapists
Higher Education Academy (HEA)	The Higher Education Academy (2011). *The UK Professional Standards Framework for teaching and supporting learning in higher education*. York: HEA.	Generic Higher Education
World Federation for Medical Education (WFME)	World Federation for Medical Education (2015). *Basic Medical Education WFME Global standards for Quality Improvement*. WFME: Ferney-Voltaire and Copenhagen.	Doctors
World Health Organisation (WHO)	World Health Organisation. (2014). *Midwifery Educator Core Competencies*. Retrieved from: https://www.who.int/hrh/nursing_midwifery/midwifery_educator_core_competencies.pdf?ua=1	Midwives
World Health Organisation (WHO)	World Health Organisation. (2016). *Nurse Educator Core Competencies*. Retrieved from: https://apps.who.int/iris/bitstream/handle/10665/258713/9789241549622-eng.pdf;jsessionid=B44ED17ECA84A88F6995995A22310A32?sequence=1	Nurses
World Federation of Occupational Therapists	World Federation of Occupational Therapists. *Minimum Standards for the Education of Occupational Therapists*. Retrieved from: https://www.wfot.org/assets/resources/COPYRIGHTED-World-Federation-of-Occupational-Therapists-Minimum-Standards-for-the-Education-of-Occupational-Therapists-2016a.pdf	Occupational Therapists

Appendix 2: Definition of Initial Codes

Assessment and Feedback	
Purpose and Methods of assessment	Range of methods to assess learners, methods appropriate for purpose. e.g., 'uses a basic range of methods to assess learners' (AoME 2014) 'Differentiate between formative and summative functions of assessment and define their role in medical education' (Academy of Medical Royal Colleges 2009)
Development of assessment	Designs/develops assessments, contributes to construction of assessments. e.g., 'Contributes to the construction of assessment items' (AoME 2014) 'Leads the strategic development and implementation of assessment processes and systems, encouraging and supporting colleagues and learners to be actively engaged' (COPDEND 2013).
Feedback	Provides effective feedback to learners, understands feedback methods and understands importance of feedback. e.g., 'Provides effective feedback to learners using a range of methods' (AoME 2014) 'Feedback following assessment must be learner centred, timely and linked to the assessment outcomes' (AHCS 2018).

(Cont'd.)

Assessment and Feedback	
Quality of assessment	Contributes to and maintains quality of assessments through continuous monitoring and improvement. e.g., *"Is aware that assessment practices require continuous monitoring and improvement"* (AoME 2014) *"Revises the curriculum based on assessment of program outcomes, learner needs, and societal and health care trends"* (Christensen & Simmons, 2020)
Learner progression	Supports and monitors progress of learner to achieve learning objectives. e.g., *"Assess progress in order to plan for the students' increasing level of skill acquisition"* (WHO 2014)' *'monitors progress of the learner in relation to planned learning outcomes"* (ANTS 2010)
Designing Education	
Evaluation of educational activity	Evaluates learning programmes, seeks and responds to feedback about own teaching and education programmes. e.g., *"evaluates and improves educational interventions"* (AoME 2014) *"The programme must have regular and effective monitoring and evaluation systems in place"* (HCPC 2017).
Learning and teaching methods, resources	Aware of a range of methods and resources for teaching and how to use effectively when planning courses. e.g., *"Is aware of a range of learning methods, experiences and resources and how they may be used effectively"* (AoME 2014). *"The best teachers are skilful with a variety of instructional activities. They are interested in learning new techniques and strategies"* (Turner, Palazzi & Ward 2008).
Learning and teaching principles	Aware of different ways of teaching and learning and applies this in design of education. e.g., *"Shows how the principles of learning and teaching are incorporated into educational developments"* (AoME 2014) *"Can describe how different ideas about learners and learning make a difference to educational practice"* (COPDEND 2013)
Learning needs	Understands the learning needs of students e.g., *"shows how the needs of learners are considered"* (AoME 2014) *"The learning, teaching and assessment methods utilise a range of techniques and technologies to address the pedagogic needs of the student body"* (College of Occupational Therapists 2014).

Designing Education	
Learning outcomes	Defines appropriate learning outcomes and what it is that is to be learned. e.g., *"Constructs appropriate learning outcomes that can be measured or judged"* (AoME 2014) *"Setting and monitoring achievement of realistic learning objectives"* (NMC 2008).
Educational Management and Leadership	
Governance	Quality assurance, development of standards/frameworks. e.g., *"Understands the roles and responsibilities of statutory and other regulatory bodies in the provision and quality assurance of medical education"* (AoME 2014) *"Contributes to educational policy and development at local or national levels"* (Academy of Medical Royal Colleges 2009).
Leadership	Leads educational teams/projects, influence beyond own organisation and influences policy. e.g., *"Leads educational projects or programmes locally"* (AoME 2014) *"Makes educational strategies explicit and guides other teachers to reflect on and use them"* (Walsh et al 2015).
Engagement with stakeholders	Engages with a range of stakeholders in order to manage and deliver educational programmes. e.g., *"Communicate best practice in nursing education with peers, students and other stakeholders"* (WHO 2016) *"Familiarizes him or herself with stakeholders' expectations (e.g. university, CFPC, province)"* (Walsh et al 2015).
Management	Manages educational programmes and resources. e.g., *"Manages educational programmes and resources, including individuals and/or financial resources at a local level"* (AoME 2014) *"Demonstrates ability to design and manage a course of study, with appropriate use of teaching, assessment and study methods"* (RPS 2013).
Cost effectiveness	Manages educational programmes and resources in a cost-effective manner. e.g., *'Devise and deliver an appropriate, cost-effective teaching programme, which promotes their ability to learn and succeed'* (The College of Social Work 2013). *'Demonstrate effective and efficient human and financial resource management'* (WHO 2016).

(Cont'd.)

Educational Scholarship and Research	
Evidence based healthcare education	Applies research evidence to teaching practice. e.g., 'Is aware of literature relevant to current developments in medical education' (AoME 2014) 'We take responsibility for advancing the professionalism and scholarship of medical education' (AMEE)
Quality improvement, innovation in HPE	Uses knowledge and research to inform and improve practice. e.g., 'Interprets and applies the results of educational research to his or her educational practice' (AoME 2014) 'Disseminate key messages / ideas fostered through practice supervision in order to benefit the MDT, clients, patients and the public' (British Dietetic Association 2013).
Teaching, Facilitating Learning, Supporting Learners	
Facilitation of Learning (Delivery of teaching)	Uses a range of educational methods and technologies to achieve learning outcomes. e.g., 'Appropriately uses a broad range of educational methods and technologies to achieve intended learning outcomes' (AoME 2014) 'provide a range of opportunities to maximise learning and enable the achievement of directed and self-directed level-appropriate learning outcomes' (HCPC 2016).
Encourages active learning	Involves learner in actual clinical experience. e.g., 'Describes ways of involving learners in actual clinical practice e.g. experiential learning opportunities' (AoME 2014) 'Appreciate the transition from a passive to an active technique and the shift of focus from teacher to student' (Turner, Palazzi & Ward 2008).
Learner reflection	Aware of importance of and encourages learners to engage in reflective practice. e.g., Uses systems of teaching and training that incorporate reflective practice in self and others' (AoME 2014) 'Demonstrate how to develop reflective skills with a learner' (CODP 2009).
Safe and effective learning environment	Establishing a safe and effective learning environment. e.g., Is aware of the importance of establishing a safe and effective learning environment' (AoME 2014) 'Providing students with adequate facilities, supervision, access to clients/patients in order that HCPC standards and BDA curriculum requirements are met' (British Dietetic Association 2013).

Values	
1 Selflessness	Holders of public office should act solely in terms of the public interest. (Committee on Standards in Public Life 1995) *e.g., 'Altruism: Overt behaviour that reflects concern for the welfare and well-being of others and assumes the responsibility of placing the needs of the patients or clients ahead of the professionals' interest' (CAIPE 2017).*
2 Integrity	Holders of public office must avoid placing themselves under any obligation to people or organisations that might try inappropriately to influence them in their work. They should not act or take decisions in order to gain financial or other material benefits for themselves, their family or their friends. They must declare and resolve any interests and relationships. (Committee on Standards in Public Life 1995). *e.g., 'The medical teaching profession sets itself demanding standards. We act with judgement, integrity and respect to build the trust and confidence of all the stakeholders including the public, the government, the healthcare professions and the learners (AMEE).*
3 Objectivity	Holders of public office must act and take decisions impartially, fairly and on merit, using the best evidence and without discrimination or bias. (Committee on Standards in Public Life 1995). *e.g., 'All staff involved in the assessment of students – formative or summative – must be informed about their link to the standards of proficiency and, where appropriate, trained to facilitate these assessments' (CORU 2017).*
4 Accountability	Holders of public office are accountable to the public for their decisions and actions and must submit themselves to the scrutiny necessary to ensure this. (Committee on Standards in Public Life 1995). *e.g., 'You are personally accountable for your professional practice and must always be prepared to justify your decisions and actions' (GMC 2015).*
5 Openness	Holders of public office should act and take decisions in an open and transparent manner. Information should not be withheld from the public unless there are clear and lawful reasons for so doing. (Committee on Standards in Public Life 1995). *e.g., 'Recommends that that the clinical curriculum is presented in an accessible and transparent manner to all students and their clinical supervisors including clearly defined objectives and methods of assessment' (INMED).*

(Cont'd.)

Values	
6 Honesty	Holders of public office should be truthful. (Committee on Standards in Public Life 1995). e.g., *'Act with honesty and integrity in relationships with patients, families, communities, and other team members'* (IPEC 2016).
7 Leadership	Holders of public office should exhibit these principles in their own behaviour. They should actively promote and robustly support the principles and be willing to challenge poor behaviour wherever it occurs. (Committee on Standards in Public Life 1995). e.g., *'Actively challenges poor practice and champions positive change in themselves and others'* (Royal College of Surgeons of Edinburgh 2017).
Equity in admissions	Fairly and appropriately selects learners for admission to a programme of study. e.g., *'Where involved in recruitment, fairly and appropriately selects learners for educational programmes'* (COPDEND 2013) *'The mechanism for student admission to the programme ensures that the stated entry requirements are met. The mechanism and conditions for students exiting the educational programme before completion are explicit and are met'* (NMBI 2016).
Context of practice	Recognises unique needs of specific area of practice. e.g., *'Recognise the unique needs of practice and contribute to development of an environment that supports achievement of NMC standards of proficiency'* (NMC 2015) *'The education provider will have a set of requirements for the selection of practice placements to ensure quality learning experiences for students that reflect the normal context and environment of practice'* (CORU 2017).
Diversity	Respect for diversity, equality of opportunity. e.g., *'Actively promotes and respects diversity in discharging his or her educational responsibilities'* (AoME 2014) *'Embrace the cultural diversity and individual differences that characterize patients, populations, and the health team'* (IPEC 2016).
Ethical	Acts in an ethical way, respects rules/laws. e.g., *'Nurse educators demonstrate professionalism including legal, ethical and professional values as a basis for developing nursing education policies, procedures and decision making'* (WHO 2016) *'embodies the Nursing Code of Conduct and Ethics in all aspect of education and practice'* (ANTS 2010).

Values	
Inspiring	Inspires students to learn and achieve learning outcomes, inspires other teachers/colleagues. e.g., *'Effective role models will inspire, teach by example, and stimulate admiration and emulation'* (BMA 2006). *'The best teachers are dynamic, exciting and stimulating. They are enthusiastic, challenging, inspiring, and motivating. They are friendly and nonthreatening. They are objective, fair, and supportive. The strongest teacher is the one who leads the learner to solve the problem and inspires the learner'* (Turner, Palazzi & Ward 2008).
Learner wellbeing	Shows concern for the wellbeing of learners. e.g., *'Acts with due consideration for the emotional, physical and psychological wellbeing of learners'* (AoME 2014) *'Psychological safety of the learner is considered and is appropriately supported'* (ASPIH).
Patient safety, quality of care	Ensures patient safety and high levels of care at all times. e.g., *'1. Ensures the safety of patients at all times 2. Promotes high quality clinical care 3. Works within appropriate clinical governance and risk management frameworks'* (AoME 2014) *'Training programmes must support safe, effective, patient centred and compassionate care at all times'* (AHCS 2018).
Personal development, reflective practice in self	Is committed to continuous personal development and reflects on own practice. e.g., *'Demonstrates willing to advance own educational capability through continuous learning'* (Academy of Medical Royal Colleges 2009) *'Demonstrate willingness to participate in professional development activities to increase performance effectiveness'* (WHO 2016).
Person-centred	Takes a person-centred approach to teaching practice. e.g., *'all learners should have an inclusive, learning-centred, empowering and level appropriate learning experience'* (HCPC 2016) *'Adopts a learner centred approach and values education and training as part of the core of clinical care'* (South Australia Medical Association 2017).

(Cont'd.)

Values	
Professional qualification, experience	Has a professional qualification or personal experience in the area in which they are teaching. e.g., *'A medical trainer is an appropriately trained and experienced doctor who is responsible for the education and training of medical students and/ or postgraduate medical trainees which takes place in an environment of medical practice'* (GMC 2012) *'Educators are required to demonstrate advanced professional practice competencies dependent on their context of educational practice'* (ANTS 2010).
Respect for learners	Demonstrates respect for learners and is committed to supporting the personal and professional development of learners. e.g., *'Respect for learners: 1. Acts with due consideration for the emotional, physical and psychological wellbeing of learners 2. Supports learners in their personal and professional development'* (AoME 2014) *'Respect and value the uniqueness and diversity of learners and recognise and build on their strengths, and take into account individual learning styles and preferred assessment methods'* (The College of Social Work 2013).
Role-Model	Acts as a role model for learners and other professionals/ teachers. e.g., *'The best teachers act as role models—from washing their hands before examining a patient to drawing out the history from an upset patient or confused parent. They help learners develop their clinical reasoning skills, as well as increase their fund of knowledge'* (Turner, Palazzi & Ward 2008). *'A good mentor from the student perspective is someone who is supportive, acts as a good role model, teacher, guide, and assessor; generally, someone who has a genuine concern and has the student's interests at heart'* (CODP 2009).
Teamwork, respect for colleagues, interprofessional practice	Works as part of a team, across professions and has respect for colleagues. e.g., *'Supports inter-, trans- and multi-professional education, learning with, from and about other professionals to improve collaborative care'* (AoME 2014) *'Training works best as a team effort. As long as the training co-ordinator/officer retains oversight, there is nothing to prevent trainees being coached and mentored in particular skills, procedures etc. by a competent, less senior member of staff. Less senior staff may also be involved in assessing the trainee's competence, provided there is quality control from the training officer. However, trainees should not assess other trainees'* (National School of Healthcare Science)

Values	
Willingness to teach, enthusiasm for teaching	The individual is willing and/or enthusiastic about teaching. *e.g., 'The quality teacher wants to teach and is prepared to take the time to do so. For the busy clinician, time is money, and the willingness to take the time to teach is a testament to the commitment of the successful clinician-educator (Turner, Palazzi & Ward 2008). 'Demonstrates willing to teach trainees and other healthcare and social care workers in a variety of settings to maximise effective communication and practical skills and to improve patient care' (Academy of Medical Royal Colleges 2009).*

Appendix 3: Coding Frequency for all Nodes

Total number of sources coded = 48

Code	Frequency
Teamwork, respect for colleagues, interprofessional practice	40
Personal development, reflective practice in self	38
Patient safety, quality of care	36
Professional qualification, experience	36
Accountability	35
Openness	34
Objectivity	32
Learning and teaching principles	30
Learning needs	30
Leadership	30
Diversity	30
Learning and teaching methods, resources	29
Integrity	28
Learner wellbeing	28

(Cont'd.)

Code	Frequency
Learning outcomes	27
Encourages reflection in learners	27
Purpose and methods of assessment	27
Feedback	26
Evidence based healthcare education	26
Safe and effective learning environment	25
Role model	25
Evaluation of educational activity	24
Governance	24
Leadership	24
Management	23
Respect for learners	23
Facilitation of learning (Delivery of teaching)	22
Quality improvement, innovation in HPE	21
Active learning	20
Ethical	20
Learner progression	16
Honesty	16
Development of assessment	16
Selflessness	14
Equity in admissions	11
Person-centred	11
Quality of assessment	10
Inspiring	10
Engagement with stakeholders	9
Willingness to teach, enthusiasm for teaching	9
Context of practice	5
Cost effectiveness	4

Appendix 4: List of Abbreviations

Acronym	Name
ACP	The Association of Child Psychotherapists
AHCS	Academy for Healthcare Science
AMEE	Association for Medical Education in Europe
AoMRC	Academy of Medical Royal Colleges
AMS	The Academy of Medical Sciences
ANTS	The Australian Nurse Teachers' Society
AoME	The Academy of Medical Educators
ASME	Association for the Study of Medical Education
ASPiH	Association for Simulated Practice in Healthcare
BASW	British Association of Social Workers
BDA	British Dietetic Association
BMA	British Medical Association
CAIPE	Centre for the Advancement of Interprofessional Education
CanMEDS	Canadian Medical Education Directives for Specialists
CFPC	The College of Family Physicians of Canada
CODP	College of Operating Department Practitioners
COPDEND	Committee of Postgraduate Dental Deans and Directors

(Cont'd.)

Acronym	Name
CORU	Health and Social Professions Council in Ireland
COT	College of Occupational Therapists
CP	College of Paramedics
CPD	Continuing Professional Development
CSP	Chartered Society of Physiotherapy
CSW	The College of Social Work
CUREMeDE	Cardiff Unit for Research and Evaluation in Medical and Dental Education
DVA	Descriptors of Values and Activities
EBMA	European Board of Medical Assessors
EBE	Evidence Based Education
EBP	Evidence Based Practice
FMLM	Faculty of Medical Leadership and Management
GDC	General Dental Council
GMC	General Medical Council
GPhC	General Pharmaceutical Council
HCE	Healthcare Educator
HCPC	Health and Care Professions Council
HCPs	Healthcare Professions
HEA	Higher Education Academy (AdvanceHE)
UKPSF	UK Professional Standards Framework
HEE	Health Education England
HEIW	Health Education and Improvement Wales
HENW	Health Education North West
HEVAS	Health Educators Values and Activities Study
HPE	Health Professions Education
ICM	International Confederation of Midwives
INHED	Irish Network of Medical Educators
INHWE	International Network for Health Workforce Education
INMED	Irish Network of Medical Educators
IPE	Interprofessional Education
IPEC	Interprofessional Education Collaborative
IPL	Interprofessional Learning
NIMDTA	Northern Ireland Medical & Dental Training Agency
NLN	National League for Nursing

Acronym	Name
NMBI	Nursing and Midwifery Board Ireland
NMC	Nursing and Midwifery Council
NScHS	National School of Healthcare Science
ODPs	Operating department practitioner
QAA	Quality Assurance Agency for Higher Education
RCN	Royal College of Nursing
RCPSC	Royal College of Physicians and Surgeons of Canada
RCS	Royal College of Surgeons
RPS	Royal Pharmaceutical Society
UKCP	UK Council for Psychotherapy
WFME	World Federation for Medical Education
WFOT	World Federation of Occupational Therapists
WHO	World Health Organisation

Index

A

Abbreviations   149
Academy of Medical Educators
   (AoME)   14, 21, 24
   *Professional Standards for
   Medical, Dental and
   Veterinary Educators*
   (2014)   14, 29, 30, 32, 33
Academy of Medical Sciences,
   Redressing the Balance
   guidelines   37, 38
Accountability   74, 76, 141
Accreditation of Interprofessional
   Health Education
   (AIPHE)   105
Active learning   44, 140
Activities   32, 106
   phase 2 of study   32, 35
   phase 3 of study
      see phase 3 (nominal group).
   phase 4 of study   53
   phase 5 of study
      see phase 5 (Delphi study).
   shared by interprofessional
      educators   xvi, 3, 11, 111
   vs values, ambiguity   98, 101
   see also descriptors of values and
      activities (DVAs).
Adverse events   3, 6
   collective responsibility of team   4
Aims of research   13
Assessment   113
   development of   44, 137
   learner progression activity, in
      phase 5   81
   methods   113, 137
   purpose   137
   quality of   44, 138
   relationship with learning and
      teaching   44
Assessment and learner
      progression   81
   relationship with learning and
      teaching
   see also learner progression.

Association for Medical Education in Europe   21
Association for Simulated Practice in Healthcare   25
Association for the Study of Medical Education   21
Attitudes   2, 11
  change needed   6, 9
Audiology/audiologists   19, 28

B

Blame, culture of   4

C

CAIPE (Centre of the Advancement of Interprofessional Education)   7, 106
Candour, duty of   5, 100
Cardiff University Research Ethics Committee   15
Career (as healthcare educator)   2, 3, 12
  career paths   114
  development   2, 3, 10
    challenges/difficulties   9, 12, 113
    core curriculum on education for all students   111
    early start to   112
    early   112
    development of material   97
Clinical error/adverse events   3, 6
  collective responsibility of team   4
Clinical practice   3, 9, 12, 116
Clinical skills centre   7
Clinical supervision   96
Clinician, transition to healthcare educator   9, 10
Codes
  analysis of standards/guidance documents   28, 29, 30, 33
  definitions for   29, 137
  frequency   33, 147

Collaboration, between health professions   7, 10, 74
Collective leadership   99
College of Social Work   37, 38
Committee on Standards in Public Life (Nolan Committee)   29, 141, 142, 143, 144, 145
Communication
  barriers, interprofessional teams   6, 9
  effective, lacking   6, 41
  failure   4, 6
    reasons   6
  improving, in teams   7, 8
  inter-group, in interprofessional education   108
  phase 3 of study   41, 43
  phase 5 of study   100
  social   5
Competence/competency
  collective (team)   5, 110
  interprofessional educators   11
  to teach   107
  to teach in interprofessional teams   9
Consensus (in Delphi study)   92, 96, 106, 115
  activities   92, 106
  criteria   71
  values   92, 98
Context of practice   41, 142
Continuing professional development (CPD)   11, 96
COPDEND *Professional Standards for Dental Educators*   35, 36
Cost effectiveness   139
Cost management   79
Culture of blame
Curriculum
  core, on education for all students   111
  hidden   10, 112
  interprofessional learning as part   12

D

Data collection, outline   15
Defensive behaviour, reducing   5
Delivery of teaching   52
Delphi method/study   15, 29, 49, 71
  interprofessional learning as part
  see also phase 5 (Delphi study).
Dentist/dentistry   19
Descriptors of values and activities (DVAs)   95
  conceptualising   100
  descriptive vs aspirational   97
  development/presentation,
    leadership debate   99
  domain groupings   102, 104
  interprofessional educators
    see also domain(s).
  employer vs individual   100
  implications of HEVA study   106
  individual vs collective
    leadership   99
  key principles   97, 98, 99, 100
  knows vs does   98
  organisational structure   101, 102
  value or activity, item as   98, 101
Diversity   50, 142
  commonality vs   50, 106
  learning needs   xvi
Domain(s)
  descriptors of values and
    activities   101
    educator progression   104
    groupings   102, 104
    organisational structure
      101, 102
    educational   xvi
Duty of candour   5, 100

E

Education
  core curriculum for health
    profession students   111
  designing   138, 139
  management   139
  valued highly as service
    delivery   48
  see also healthcare education;
    interprofessional education.
Educational activity, evaluation   138
Educational domains   xvi
Educational excellence   114
Educational theory and
  practice   96, 97
Education system
  see healthcare education system.
Educators
  broad term, description   47
  importance of role   47
  personal development as   74
  progression   104
  see also healthcare educators
    (HCEs); interprofessional
    educators.
Employer vs individual   99
Engagement with others   46
Enhancing quality (phase 5 activity)
  see quality, enhancing.
Enthusiasm for teaching   145
Equity in admissions   98, 142
Errors, preventable   3
  guilt relating to   4
  prevention, effective team work   5
Ethical conduct   74
Ethical responsibility, healthcare
  educators   100
Ethics   142
Evidence base, for professionalising
  healthcare education   114
Evidence-based healthcare
  education   140

F

Fairness
  in admissions   98, 142
  value in phase 3 of study   41, 43, 47
  value in phase 5 of study   74

Federation of healthcare
    education   1, 116
Feedback   44, 74, 83, 87, 137
  student   28
Francis report/Mid Staffordshire
    Inquiry   5
Funding   40
Future perspectives   40, 46, 116

G

General Medical Council   21, 24, 25
General practice   3
Governance   139
Guidelines for training   2
Guilt, after medical error   4

H

Harm, in primary care   4
  collective responsibility of team   4
  frequency   3
Health and care Professions
    Council   21, 41
Healthcare education
  as a discipline   11, 113
  challenges to   116
  concern over standards   111
  defining excellence in   113
  failure, tribalism   2, 105
  individual professions
    competence and standards
      maintained   107
    transmission model, educator to
      learner   107, 108
  professional bodies in   12, 13
  professionalising   11, 113
  requirements   114
  role model   113
  status of a discipline lacking   113
Healthcare education community   1
Healthcare education
    organisations   1
Healthcare education system   7

current limitations   7
designed for results achieved   7
interprofessional
    see Interprofessional
    education (IPE).
Healthcare educators (HCEs)
  activities, HEVA study
    see activities.
  clinicians as; cliniciansas   9, 112
  commonality and divergence   11,
    50, 106
  competency to teach   107
  educational skills   10, 112
  ethical responsibility   100
  from smaller professions   95
  from specific professions, unique
    skills/values   115
  HEVA study phase 3
    participants   40
  improving, core curriculum on
    education for students   111
  individual *vs* employer, roles   99
  initial appointment   10
  interprofessional
    see interprofessional educators.
  interprofessional teams
    see interprofessional teams, of
    educators.
  leadership, collective *vs*
    individual   99
  outstanding   113
  professional identity acquisition   10
  quality enhancement   103
  reluctant teachers   112
  reward system failure   9
  role lacking recognition   2, 9, 12
  senior, leadership   99
  shared activities/values   xvi, 3,
    11, 111
  shared generic skills   11, 115
  standards for
    see standards and guidance
    documents.

support for   3, 13
  interprofessional   13
training
  see training of healthcare educators.
transition from clinician to   9, 10
transition to interprofessional
    educator   10, 12
  challenges   12
work, holistic view   2
Healthcare Educators Values and
    Activities (HEVA)
  see HEVA study.
Healthcare professionals (HCPs)
  CPD, educational
  early start to educator identity
    development   112
  educational role   9, 112
    transition from clinician
      to   9, 10
  educational theory/practice
    training   96, 97
  professionalising education   11, 113
  representation in HEVA study   95
  supervision, assessment and
    mentoring roles   96
Health Education and Improvement
    Wales (HEIW)   13, 15
Health Education England
    (HEE)   13, 15, 25
  standards documents   28
HEVA study   111, 112, 115
  aims; aims   13
  challenges as a result of   116
  conclusions   104
  dynamic interaction, educator
    progression   104
  high level training of healthcare
    educators   114, 115
  implications and outcome   106
  limitations; limitations   96, 106
  phases
    *see individual phases
    (under Phase)*.

rationale and background   15
  skills for interprofessional
    educators   115
  team for   96
  see also activities; descriptors of
    values and activities (DVAs);
    values, professional.
Hidden curriculum   10, 112
Hierarchies, failure of teamworking
    due to   6
Higher Education
    Academy   21, 25
Higher Education
    Authority   21, 24
Holistic view, work of healthcare
    educators   2
Honesty   142

I

Identity, professional, as educator
  acquisition   10
  early start to   112
  not shared with learners,
    interprofessional
    educators   109
  shared   111
INHWE (International Network
    for Health Workforce
    Education)   15, 49, 72, 100
Innovation   40, 46
Innovative methods   87
Inspiring, value   143
Integrity   141
International Network for Health
    Workforce Education
    (INHWE)   15, 49, 72, 100
Interprofessional education
    (IPE)   8, 15
  as activity *vs* a value   98
  as value, phase 5 of study   74
    Round 2 results   89, 90
  common educational
    language   114

common framework for improvements   111
common understanding of what is shared   114
definition   7, 107
future prospects   116
improving, requirements   113
model, complexity   108
overlap between professions   111
tasks   8
teams and facilitators involved   8, 109, 110
transition from clinician to
see also interprofessional teams, of educators.
to improve patient safety   7
Interprofessional educators   8, 106
additional skills needed   115
authenticity, credibility and communication   109
competency to teach   107
complexity of role   108, 110
profession not shared with learners   109
team of educators and learners   8, 109, 110
identity development   112
identity revised, shared values/activities   111
shared professional identity   111
team of
see interprofessional teams.
training needs of   8
transition from educator to   10, 12
challenges   12
Interprofessional federation of healthcare education organisations   116
Interprofessional learning (IPL)   xv, 12, 106
as key part of curricula   12
complexities   110
in phase 3 of study   41, 43
Interprofessional practice   43, 144

Interprofessional teaching   xvi
complexities   110
see also interprofessional educators.
Interprofessional teams, of
educators   8, 9, 109, 110, 116
barriers to communication   6, 9
competency   9, 11
improving   7
complexity of role   108, 110
staff development   7, 9
see also team(s); teamworking.
Ireland   40

K

Knowledge   106
clinical, each profession   2, 11
educational theory   96
Knows vs does   98

L

Leadership   41, 99, 139, 142
as value or activity   98
dimensions of   99
individual vs collective   99
Learner(s)
reflection   140
respect for   74
wellbeing   143
Learner progression   83, 97, 101, 138
activities included   81
comments by participants   83
consensus; consensus   92
Round 1 rating   81, 82
Learning
active, encouraging   140
by professionals   6, 7
facilitation   140
needs   138
preparation for
see preparation for teaching and learning.

resources 78, 138
social 8
supporting
 see teaching and supporting learning.
 teaching and assessment relationship 44
Learning and teaching principles 138
Learning environment 101, 140
Learning needs, diversity, interprofessional group xvi
Learning outcomes 77, 78
Literature review 28, 99
Litigation 4

M

Management, education 139
Mid Staffordshire NHS Foundation Hospital Trust 5
Multidisciplinary team (healthcare)
 effective working 5
 responsibility for patient safety 5
Multiprofessional education 8
 responsibility for patient safety
 see also interprofessional education (IPE).

N

NHS
 Five Year Forward View – Next Steps 105
 Long Term Plan 105
Nominal group process 39
Nurses 19
Nursing and Midwifery Council 21, 24
 Standards to Support Learning and Assessment in Practice 35, 36
NVivo software 14, 28, 35

O

Objectivity 141
Occupational therapy/therapists 19
Openness 141
Optometry/optometrists 19, 28

P

Patient care 4, 11, 79, 100, 112
Patient involvement in health education 41
Patient safety 7, 143
 common language for professionals 11
 healthcare educator responsibility 100
 improving interprofessional communication 7
 improving team working to enhance 7
 role of teams 4, 11
 upholding 74
Patient wellbeing, upholding 74
Personal development, as educator 74, 87, 143
Personal qualities, 'unmeasurable' 50
Person-centred approach 143
Pharmacy/pharmacists 19
Phase 1 (initial survey) 14, 25
 appraisal of educator practice 21, 22
 method 18
 professional organisations for educators 20, 21
 membership by respondents 19, 20, 21
 purpose 17
 recruitment 14
 regulatory organisations 21, 22
 respondents, and roles 18, 19, 25
 responsibility to regulatory body 21
 results 24
 standards/guidelines for practice 22, 23, 24, 25

standards for appraisal as
  educators   21, 23, 24, 25
Phase 2 (analysis of standards/
  guidance documents)   14, 38
  activities   32, 35
  analysis method   30, 33
  AoMS and College of Social Work
    standards comparison   37, 38
  codes used   28, 29, 30, 33
    definitions for   29, 137
  core activities   35
  differences in content of
    documents   33, 34
  findings   33, 147
  initial survey   28, 33
  literature review   28, 99
  methods   28
  NMC and COPDEND standards
    comparison   35, 36
  professional values/qualities   31,
    33, 35
    variations   35
  standards documents
    analysed   28, 129
  summary of findings   33
Phase 3 (nominal group)   14, 48, 72
  activities   45, 47, 100
    amended, first round voting   46
    amended, second round
      voting   47
  current issues for educators   41
  nominal group process   39
  participants   40, 48
  results   47
  summary of findings   48
  values and personal qualities   42,
    43, 100
    amended, first round voting   43
    amended, second round
      voting   43, 44
Phase 4 (workshop)   15, 70
  activities   53
  methods   49

results   70
  by group   70
  subgroups, traits   53, 70
  values/principles   50, 51
    commonality and diversity
      50, 106
Phase 5 (Delphi study)   15, 93
  activities   87
    consensus (final)   92, 106
    enhancing quality   87, 103
    learner progression   83, 101
    preparation for teaching/
      learning   77, 78, 79, 101
    Round 1 list   76
    Round 1 results   87
    Round 2 list   88
    Round 2 results   90, 91, 92
    teaching and supporting
      learning   81, 101
    working in teams   85
    see also individual activities.
  consensus criteria   71
  Delphi process   71
  domain groupings   102, 104
  final consensus   92, 96, 106, 115
  participants   73
  recruitment   72
  Round 1   89
    conclusions   89
    final comments   87, 88
    participants   73
    results   89
  Round 2   89, 92
    results   92
  rounds of survey   72
  values   74, 101
    central   101
    comments   76
    items as values *vs* activities   98
    Round 1 list   74
    Round 1 results   75, 76
    Round 2 list   88
    Round 2 results   89, 90

Physiotherapy/physiotherapists   19
Policy development   40
Preparation for teaching and
    learning   78, 101
  activities included   77
  comments by participants   78
  consensus   92
  Round 1 rating   77, 78
Preparedness for futures   46, 47
Primary discipline   12, 114
Professional identity as educator
    see identity, professional,
    as educator.
Professionalism   11, 41, 113
Professional organisations for
    educators   20, 21
  membership by HEVA
      respondents   19, 20, 21
  see also specific organisations.
Professional qualifications   43, 144
Professional Standards Authority,
    UK   105
Programme Governance   100

Q

Qualification, professional   43
Quality, enhancing (phase 5)   87, 103
  activities included   85
  comments by participants   87
  consensus   92
  Round 1 rating   85, 86
Quality, in education   74
Quality improvement, code   140
Quality of care   143

R

Recognition of educator role   3, 11,
    47, 113
  lacking   2, 9, 12
Reflective practice   140, 143
Regulators/regulatory body   21, 22
  interprofessional education   108

monitoring graduates   107
  responsibility to   21
Resources, teaching/learning
    78, 138
Respect
  for colleagues   74, 144
  for learners   74, 144
Role-model   144
Royal Pharmaceutical Society (RPS),
    standards documents   28

S

Safe learning environment   79, 140
Safety management systems   4
Second victim, concept   4
Selflessness   141
Seven principles of public life,
    The (1995)   29
Shared values/activities   xvi, 3,
    11, 111
Simulation, team-based   7
Skills
  clinical, centre   7
  educational   10, 112
  shared generic, healthcare
      educators   11, 115
  taken for granted   47
Social causes, failure to teams to
    work together   6
Social communication   5
Social learning   8
Social media, recruitment for
    research   14, 18
  phase 5 (Delphi study)   72
Stakeholders, engagement with   139
Standards (professional)   113
  appraisal of educators   21, 23, 24, 25
  publicly available, to professionalise
      healthcare education   113
  relevance, appreciating   47
  shared/common, interprofessional
      educators   114

Standards and guidance
    documents 95
  analysis
    see phase 2.
  for individuals vs employing
      institutions 99
  literature review 28, 99
  phase 1 (initial survey) 22, 23,
      24, 25
Student(s)
  core curriculum on
      education 111
  feedback 28
Study
  see HEVA study.
Supervision 96
Supervisors, educational and
    clinical 10
Survey, initial, HEVA study
  see phase 1 (initial survey).

T

Teachers
  healthcare
    see healthcare educators
        (HCEs).
  non-clinical 9
Teaching
  delivery 140
  interprofessional teams
    see interprofessional educators;
        interprofessional teams, of
        educators.
  principles 138
  resources 78, 138
Teaching and supporting
    learning 81, 97, 101
  activities included 79
  comments by participants 81
  consensus 92
  Round 1 rating, results 79, 80
Team(s)
  communication, barriers 6, 9

competence 5, 110
  failure to work together 6
  interprofessional
    see interprofessional teams, of
        educators.
  junior members, concerns 6
  role, talking about mistakes 4
  role in safe patient care
      provision 4
Teamwork
  value, in phase 2 of
      study 30, 35
  value, in phase 3 of study 43
Teamworking
  change in attitudes needed 6
  complexity 8
  democratic approach to 6
  essential for patient safety 11
  failure, harm to patients 4
  improving communication 7
  improving to enhance patient
      safety 7
  phase 5 activity 85
    activities included 83, 89
    comments by participants 85
    consensus 92
    Round 1 rating results 83, 84
  skills taken for granted 47
  see also interprofessional teams.
Technology 40
Territorialism 2, 9
Threshold concept 10
To Err is Human (report, IOM
    2000) 3
Training of healthcare
    educators 12, 115
  guidelines 2
  mono-professional nature 12
  to professionalise healthcare
      education 114
Transition
  from clinician to healthcare
      educator 9, 10

from healthcare educator to interprofessional educator   10, 12
Tribalism   2, 9, 105
Trust, interprofessional education   108, 110

V

Values, professional   xvi, 106, 141, 142, 143, 144, 145
  activity *vs*, ambiguity   98, 101
  descriptors
    see descriptors of values and activities (DVAs).
  organisational structure   101
  phase 2 of study
    see phase 2 (analysis of standards/guidance documents).
  phase 3 of study
    see phase 3 (nominal group).
  phase 4 of study
    see phase 4 (workshop).
  phase 5 of study
    see phase 5 (Delphi study).
  shared   xvi, 3, 11, 111
  shared by interprofessional educators   xvi, 3, 11, 111

W

WFME *Global Standards for Quality Improvement*   28
Willingness to teach   145
Working in teams
  see teamworking.
Workshop
  see phase 4 (workshop).
World Health Organisation (2016) Nurse Educator Core Competencies   33

www.ingramcontent.com/pod-product-compliance
Lightning Source LLC
Chambersburg PA
CBHW040457240426
43665CB00039B/73